Vegan
Lunch Box
Around
the World

Vegan Lunch Box

Around the World

125 Easy, International Lunches Kids and Grown-Ups Will Love!

Jennifer McCann

Da Capo
∞
LIFE
LONG

A Member of the Perseus Books Group

Designed by Trish Wilkinson
Set in 12-point Goudy by the Perseus Books Group

Library of Congress Cataloging-in-Publication Data

McCann, Jennifer.
    Vegan lunch box around the world : 125 easy, international lunches kids and
grown-ups will love! / by Jennifer McCann.
        p.   cm.
    Includes bibliographical references and index.
    ISBN 978-0-7382-1357-6 (alk. paper)
    1. Vegan cookery. 2. Lunchbox cookery. I. Title.
TX837.M2386 2009
641.5'636—dc22   2009016235

First Da Capo Press edition 2009

Published by Da Capo Press
A Member of the Perseus Books Group
www.dacapopress.com

Da Capo Press books are available at special discounts for bulk
purchases in the U.S. by corporations, institutions, and other organizations.
For more information, please contact the Special Markets Department at the Perseus
Books Group, 2300 Chestnut Street, Suite 200, Philadelphia, PA 19103, or call
(800) 810-4145, ext. 5000, or e-mail special.markets@perseusbooks.com.

10 9 8 7 6 5 4 3 2

Acknowledgments

Thanks to all the blog followers—you guys rock! Thank you to everyone at Da Capo Press who encouraged me to write this book and helped in the process. Thanks to everyone who helped with recipes, inspirations, and testing—Elane Beach, Linda Fredrick, Heather Steach, Teresa Campbell, Casey Bell—and to Martie for the gumbo.

A great big THANK YOU to Michelle Ellis for taking all the fabulous photographs you see in this book and for being my friend and helping me eat all the food after the pictures were done. Thanks to my mom, Susan Moore, for recipe testing and for putting up with her crazy daughter for all those years. Thanks and love to my husband, Greg, and of course, to James. You'll always be my little shmoo.

Contents

Part One
The Menus

Part Two
The Recipes

Introduction

Where to next? In my first book, *Vegan Lunch Box*, my lunch box visited Ethiopia, Mexico, England, Greece, India, Thailand, and Japan. I thought that that was it—I had traveled far and said all I had to say about lunch-friendly vegan cuisine.

But after the book was finished, I kept making new lunches and hearing the call of the road: why, I hadn't visited China, or Morocco, or Turkey, or Australia! And what about all the interesting cultural cuisines of my own United States: New England, California, New York, the Southwest? There were still so many foods to try and new menus to share.

Best of all, as I took pictures of these new lunches and put them up on my Vegan Lunch Box blog (www.veganlunchbox.com), I realized that some of them were in fact the very best I had ever made. I was excited by all I was learning, and amazed at how big the world of vegan cooking really turned out to be.

Vegan Lunch Box Around the World came out of that excitement, and is all about the meals I enjoy the most: meals that are plant-based, well-balanced, healthy, and inspired by cuisines and cultures from around the world.

I believe that one of the keys to becoming a successful vegan is to *replace every food you've eliminated with something new*. This can be a brand new food or a new way to prepare an old food. That way, instead of focusing on what you can't have and perhaps feeling a bit deprived, you will be focusing on all the new tastes and flavors that you now have more room in your diet to enjoy. There are so many wonderful plant-based foods out there; vegan cooking should be a celebration of all this abundance.

Enjoy your culinary wanderings!

—*Jennifer McCann*

A Note on Cultural Authenticity

Please note that not all of these recipes are spot-on traditional. I've taken some liberties in making my recipes vegan and perhaps a bit more Western, adding new elements or eliminating hard-to-find ingredients. I've also invented some brand-new recipes inspired by the spirit of the culture I was working with.*

I've also toned down the spiciness of some of the more authentic recipes, especially in dishes from Asia and India, where the usual level of heat would be too much for most Western tongues. I'm hoping that these milder versions will appeal even to our youngest family members.

Still, it's been my goal to stay true to the spirit of the original cuisines, in hopes that these small glimpses into new, rich worlds of taste and flavor will inspire you and your family to continue your vegan culinary adventures. If you find a certain cuisine that speaks to you, keep exploring! Your local library or bookstore will have many more cookbooks specializing in these various ethnic cuisines.

---

*I've marked the recipes that are the most traditional by noting the country of origin below the recipe title.

A Note on Ingredients

I've made every effort to use ingredients that can be found in most grocery and health food stores. I also list substitutions in cases where something may be hard to find. Specialty items can usually be found online; I've suggested Web sites when possible. See the Recommended Resources section at the end of the book for more information.

That said, don't be afraid to venture into your local ethnic grocery stores. Asian, Indian, and Hispanic markets are fun places to browse around in and are a great source for new foods and fresh produce, usually at quite reasonable prices.

- **Allergies:** Since the writing of my first book allergies among schoolchildren have continued to rise, and many more school districts are instituting bans on nuts and other high-allergen foods in classrooms. In response to this I've done my best to limit the number of recipes that call for nuts, especially peanuts, and most of the time nuts are entirely optional. I've also indicated beside each recipe whether it contains other common allergens like gluten, wheat, soy, and corn. (You'll be happy to note that all vegan recipes are free of those other common allergens: milk, eggs, and seafood.)

- Whenever a traditional recipe calls for chicken- or beef-flavored broth or bouillon cubes, I've used Celifibr brand bouillon cubes. They are vegan, all-natural, gluten-free, and soy-free (they do contain corn flour). Look for them at your health food store or online at www.veganstore.com.

- I use reduced sodium soy sauce in all my recipes that call for soy sauce.

- In any recipe that calls for nondairy milk, I have used plain sweetened or unsweetened Silk brand soymilk to test the recipe. Substitute any nondairy milk you prefer—soy, rice, oat, almond, multigrain, or even light coconut.

- **How to blanch and peel tomatoes:** Many of my recipes call for peeled, diced tomatoes. Here's the easiest way to do it: bring a medium saucepan filled with water to a boil. Place whole tomatoes into the boiling water for 30 to 45 seconds. You may see the skin start to split and curl. Immediately scoop out the tomatoes and place them in a bowl filled with ice water (or do it the lazy way like me and simply rinse them quickly under cold running water until they are cool to the touch). Use a sharp knife to cut out the stem, and the skin should slip right off. Dice the tomatoes and you're all set!

QUICK AND EASY VARIATION: If blanching seems like too much of a pain, substitute canned diced tomatoes. In my recipes one large tomato, peeled and diced, equals about 1 cup drained, canned diced tomatoes.

I've included these symbols to help you navigate on your journey through this book . . .

 These recipes are exceptionally fast and simple, both in their preparation and the time it takes to put them together. Depend on these dishes on days when you know time will be short.

 These are the recipes that were the most universally popular with the kids I cooked for. Of course, that doesn't mean kids won't like the other recipes, too! These are just a good place to start.

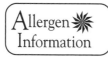 For those of you with allergies or food sensitivities, every recipe includes a note about possible allergens in the recipe as written. I've included the most common allergens in my list: gluten, wheat, soy, nuts, and corn. (Because all these recipes are vegan you never have to worry about those other common allergens—dairy, eggs, fish, and shellfish.)

How to Pack the Best Lunches Ever

PACKING A BALANCED LUNCH

Each menu in this book has been designed to provide a complete, well-balanced, vegan meal. A well-balanced lunch should include the following:

- **Vegetables (cooked or raw).** Nutrition superheroes, vegetables should be an essential part of the daily diet. Offer a rainbow of colors (orange, red, purple, and especially green) to supply your family with vitamins, minerals, and health-protecting phytochemicals.
- **Fruits (cooked, dried, frozen, or raw).** Fruit is second only to vegetables as an excellent source of vitamins, fiber, and phytochemicals. Again, offer a rainbow of colors.
- **Protein (beans, tempeh, tofu, meat analogues, etc.).** Protein is found in almost every food we eat, so lack of protein is not the big concern you might expect it to be on a vegan diet. Eat a wide

variety of healthy whole foods and include a few of these protein-rich vegan options and your protein needs are sure to be met.

- **Carbohydrates (rice, pasta, bread, etc.).** Carbs give your body energy and also help fill you up so you stay satisfied from lunchtime to the end of the work or school day. Try to eat mostly complex carbohydrates like whole wheat and brown rice.
- **Healthy fats (soy, oils, nuts and seeds, avocado, etc.).** I know fat has gotten a bad name, but including some fat in the diet is important for health, especially for young growing bodies. Nuts, seeds, and avocados are great whole food sources of healthy fats.
- **Calcium.** A single-serving tetra pack of calcium-fortified nondairy beverage is an easy way to include some calcium with every lunch. Calcium-fortified orange juice is another good choice (and contains more bioavailable calcium than cow's milk!). Other vegan sources include green vegetables (like kale, collards, and okra), quinoa, blackstrap molasses, calcium-set tofu, and almonds.
- **Water.** Pack plenty of water to drink instead of consuming the empty calories found in sweetened, carbonated beverages.

When you are packing the lunch, ask yourself

- Is the lunch nutritionally balanced?
- Do the textures and tastes work well together?
- Is the lunch colorful and attractive?

MAKING SUBSTITUTIONS

Use the guidelines above to make substitutions in the menus in the next section, switching out foods you know won't get eaten for ones that will. If all these foods are new to you, perhaps you can take the time to make one new recipe at a time and fill in the rest of the lunch with old favorites, including fast fixes like cooked frozen vegetables, a sliced apple, or baby carrots with dip. Enlist your family's help in choosing and preparing what to pack.

PACKING A SAFE LUNCH

Pack perishable foods cold and include an ice pack. Perishable foods (this includes soy foods, beans, sprouts, rice, cooked vegetables, salad dressings, etc.) should be kept cold until lunchtime. In addition to an ice pack, packing a frozen container of nondairy yogurt, applesauce, juice, or water can help keep things cold.

- Beverages sealed in unopened tetra packs, canned fruit cups, and dry foods like trail mix and pretzels will be fine without an ice pack. (Also see "Keeping Food Hot" and "Eating Things Cold" below).
- **Wash hands before handling or eating food.** It's best to wash hands with warm soapy water, but if you or your children don't have access to a sink at lunchtime, pack an individually wrapped disposable hand wipe, or do as the Japanese do and pack an *oshibori*—a small, damp washcloth packed in a plastic carrying case. Baby-size washcloths make excellent oshibori. Throw used oshibori in the laundry and wash and dry the plastic case along with your lunch box.
- **Throw away any leftovers.** Any leftover foods that weren't eaten during the day should be discarded when you get home. An ice pack can't be relied upon to keep perishable foods fresh long past lunchtime.
- **Clean all lunch bags and containers after each use.** Use hot soapy water and air dry overnight before repacking. Be sure to clean all the lunch box containers, even outer containers that hold smaller inner containers.

CHOOSING A LUNCH BOX

Here's the fun part—choosing a lunch box! There are a wide variety of lunch boxes out there to suit all your needs. I personally have a monstrous collection and recommend having at least two, so one can be in the dishwasher while you pack the other.

Here are the things to think about when choosing a lunch box:

Size

Are you packing for a kindergartner or your construction-worker husband? Do you eat sandwiches or large salads? Do you prefer one or two big dishes or lots of smaller ones? Plan accordingly and choose the size and shape that works for your eating style.

Material

I recommend reusable plastic containers for schoolchildren, as stainless steel containers dent quite easily and daily use of disposables is quite wasteful. Glass jars and containers should never be used in a child's lunch, as they are breakable.

The **Laptop Lunch System** (www.laptoplunches.com) is by far the most popular lunch box I know of for the little kid set. The colorful containers make lunch fun and attractive, so much so that they have even spawned an entire subculture of people (like me!) who take pictures of their lunches every day and share them with others over the Internet. The inner containers are cleverly held in place by the lid of the outer box; this lack of lids means fewer parts to keep track of at school.

If the Laptop is getting too small for the older kids but plastic is still in order, I recommend the new **Lunchsense** lunch box (www.lunch

sense.com) out of Eugene, Oregon. There are three different sizes to choose from (small, medium, and large), and each set comes with a beverage container, ice pack, and several individual plastic containers with tight snap-top lids. The niftiest part is that the fabric case folds out into a placemat!

The lunch boxes I prefer for myself and other adults are the stainless steel "tiffin" models like those available from **To-Go Ware** (www.to-goware.com). Stainless steel is attractive, does not absorb odors, and is better for the environment. Most of the stainless steel containers hold larger portions, perfect for those like me who like to take big salads for lunch.

Style

Let your lunch box be a reflection of your personality, something that will make you smile when you see it. Stick to something conservative and simple if you like, or go crazy! In addition to the lunch boxes noted above, there are hundreds of amazing Japanese bento (lunch) boxes available in an overwhelming array of colors, shapes, and styles. An online shop like **I Love Obento** (www.iloveobento.com) can introduce you to all the stylish possibilities.

Safety

Whichever lunch box system you choose, make sure it has the following:

- An insulated carrying case that encloses the lunch box completely.
- An ice pack or freezable lid to keep foods cold. Again, I would recommend having at least two, so the first one can have time to refreeze while you use the other.

KEEPING FOOD HOT

If you don't have access to a microwave at work or school, purchase an insulated food jar to pack any foods you wish to keep warm until lunchtime. Preheat the food jar by filling it with boiling water and letting it sit for 10 minutes before filling.

If you tend to have more than one dish that you wish to keep warm until lunchtime, consider purchasing a multicontainer insulated food jar such as the **Mr. Bento** or the **Thermos Nissan All-in-One Meal Carrier**. These insulated jars contain four separate stacking containers with lids, so you can pack several items separately and keep them all warm until mealtime.

EATING THINGS COLD

One of the biggest questions I get regarding my packed lunches is, "How does your son heat up [those vegetables, that hand pie, etc.] at lunchtime?" The answer is, he doesn't! If something definitely needs to be eaten hot I pack it in a preheated insulated food jar. Most other foods, like cooked vegetables, pot stickers, and veggie burgers, he happily eats cold.

Kids can enjoy a surprising number of foods cold that we would normally expect to eat hot. In many cases foods may even have more flavor when cool. If this sounds odd, just think about all the time you spent blowing on every bite your kids ate when they were little, trying to get their food cool enough for them to eat it.

"DO YOU HONESTLY EXPECT KIDS TO EAT ALL THIS STUFF?"

No, not all of it! Just like everyone else, each of our children is born with their unique taste preferences. You'll probably find that your children (and your spouse and yourself) like some of these recipes and don't care for others. Give every new food a try at least twice, and then move on for a while if they're not to your or your family's liking. Try leaving out ingredients you know they won't like (in my house that means no onions) or making modifications to suit their tastes.

On the other hand, I think we do a great disservice to our children when we cater too much, expecting them to like nothing but bland, junky "kid food." We as parents can't shrug our shoulders and stop offering healthy foods just because our kids would rather eat marshmallows. It breaks my heart when I hear parents dismissing healthy foods before their children even have a chance to try them, telling me, "Oh no, my kid would never eat that." Trust me, unjunk your kitchen and start offering healthy choices, and you may be surprised!

OTHER EQUIPMENT YOU WILL NEED

Along with the usual kitchen items (saucepans, cutting board, etc.), there are a few tools I highly recommend you have on hand:

- **A well-seasoned cast-iron skillet or nonstick sauté pan.** I've been able to do away with all my nonstick pans over the last two years, relying instead on my well-seasoned cast-iron skillet to sauté any food without sticking. It took a few years to season the pan to that extent, and along the way I had to depend on a nonstick pan when cooking notorious stickers like tofu or potatoes. I recommend a 10-inch skillet for most needs.
- **A powerful blender.** It's worth every penny to invest in the best blender you can afford. I have a VitaMix and use it every day, sometimes three or four times a day. It's lasted for over a decade now, and I can't imagine how many cheaper blenders I would have burned through in that time. Nothing produces a more pleasant smoothie, creamed soup, or vegan "cheese" sauce than a VitaMix.

- **A food processor.** Useful for chopping and shredding vegetables, processing beans and rice into burgers, pulsing oats into oat flour, and so on. Although not as essential as a good blender, food processors are handy in situations where a blender would process foods too finely.
- **A Microplane zester.** Sometimes I call for fresh citrus zest or grated ginger. If you don't already have one, I recommend purchasing a Microplane Zester/Grater for this. This clever tool is extremely efficient and makes quick work of the job, leaving you with perfect, delicate citrus zest and beautiful mounds of string-free ginger every time.
- **Cookie cutters.** A variety of shapes and sizes can help turn plain sandwiches, fruits, or vegetables into bite-size cuties and pretty garnishes. Small stainless steel cutters are best for cutting through fruits and vegetables (do a search online for "stainless steel vegetable cutters" and you'll find a nice assortment).

Part 1
THE MENUS

UNITED STATES

CALIFORNIA

California Roll (page 110)
Edamame (see below)
Oranges with Raspberry Sauce and
    Pickled Ginger (page 209)
Beverage: Vegan Mary (page 244)

I spent several years living in California, and two foods always come to mind when I think of it: **sushi** and **oranges**. All my favorite veggie sushi were rolled right in front of me every week by the sushi chef at my neighborhood sushi bar. Wintertime in California meant citrus trees loaded with colorful, ripe fruit and countertops at the office covered with free lemons, oranges, and grapefruits from coworkers' gardens.

Look for protein-rich frozen **edamame** (baby soybeans) in the freezer section at your local grocery store; cook them according to package directions and sprinkle with salt or garlic salt to taste.

HAWAII

PuPus (see below)
Maui Onion Dip (page 62)
Huli-Huli Tofu (page 119)
Aloha Sweet Potatoes (page 160)
Tropical Fruit Salad (page 213)

Pack a luau in your lunch box! For fun, get into the spirit of the islands and wrap your lunch bag in a plastic lei or wear a Hawaiian shirt to work or school. Top the **Tropical Fruit Salad** with a paper umbrella (trim off the sharp end if packing into a child's lunch).

PuPu means appetizer. In this case, make your appetizer a healthy one by packing an assortment of fresh vegetable crudités (carrots, celery, broccoli, sugar snap peas, etc.) with **Maui Onion Dip**. *Aloha!*

HOME SICK LUNCH

Hot Noodle Soup (page 93)
Barley Crackers (page 49)
JiggleGels (page 223)
Beverage: Lemon-Lime Sparkle (page 238)

We can't always be out adventuring at lunchtime. Everyone needs to spend a day at home now and then, curled up on the couch, recuperating with a hot bowl of soup. But don't take it out on the chickens! A vegan bowl of **Hot Noodle Soup** is just the thing—quick to make, yet soothing and flavorful.

Serve the soup with homemade crackers and a fun vegan alternative to gelatin—**JiggleGels!**

KANSAS

Mini Veggie Burgers (page 126) on
    Mini Burger Buns (page 196)
Baked frozen french fries or Tater Tots
Limeade Fruit Salad (page 207)
Oatmeal Cookies (page 227)

One of the inspirations for this cookbook was the children's book *This Is the Way We Eat Our Lunch: A Book About Children Around the World* by Edith Baer. My favorite lunchtime rhyme took place in Kansas, U.S.A.:

> "But the favorite lunch of Reggie's
> is a burger made of—VEGGIES!"

NEBRASKA

Chik'n Pot Pie (page 113)
Sticks-and-Stones Salad (page 83)
Apples with Caramel Dip (page 59)

Pies filled with savory ingredients are called "pot pies" here in the United States. The chicken pot pie was the first mass-marketed frozen pot pie, developed in 1951 by the Swanson company in Omaha, Nebraska. Frozen pot pies are still extremely popular all across the United States. This homemade vegan version is much healthier, lower in fat, and just as tasty.

NEW ENGLAND

New England Chowder (page 99)
Fish Crackers (page 53)
Boston Brown Bread Muffins (page 187)
Vegan cream cheese
A pear

A steaming bowl of **New England Chowder** is a warm, soothing comfort food for folks all along the eastern coast of the United States. You won't miss the traditional clams and cream in this recipe, with its chewy mushrooms and fresh corn "cream." Floating tiny crackers on top of the chowder is a must, and these "cheesy" little fishies are just the thing.

What ode to New England would be complete without **Boston Brown Bread**? This muffin-size version is studded with raisins and walnuts and sweetened with a touch of molasses. Spread your muffin with **vegan cream cheese** and enjoy it along with a sweet **pear** for dessert.

QUICK AND EASY VARIATION: If you don't have time to make your own cheese-flavored crackers, pick up a box of Eco-Planet Non-Dairy Cheddar Crackers. That's right, vegan cheese crackers, people! You'll find them in health food stores or online at stores like Vegan Essentials (www.veganessentials.com).

NEW ORLEANS

Martie's Gumbo (page 95)
White or brown rice
Peaches Praline (page 210)

Nothing says Louisiana like a hearty bowl of gumbo—a thick stew of tomatoes, okra, and meats (in this case, vegan sausage) served over steamed rice. Gumbo was born in New Orleans, and in it you see the various cultures of the region coming together: the traditional French bouillabaisse combining with West African okra, Spanish peppers, and Native American sassafras (*filé*).

Pralines (pronounced "PRAW-leens" in New Orleans) are caramel candies filled with chopped pecans. In this dessert a softer praline sauce makes a sweet topping for fresh sliced peaches.

NEW YORK

> Mini bagels with vegan cream cheese
> Potato Parsnip Latkes (page 174)
> Tzimmes (page 186)
> Chocolate Babka Muffins (page 217)

This menu celebrates Jewish American food culture. Immigrants to New York brought together the rich traditions of both Ashkenazi (Eastern European) and Sephardi (Mediterranean) Jewish cuisine. Many of these foods are now staples in the United States, like the **bagels** found in every grocery store. Others, like **latkes** and **babka**, are not as well known but certainly deserve to be.

PICNIC TIME

> Baguette with Roasted Red Pepper Spread (page 85)
> Picnic Potato Salad (page 82)
> Barbecue Baked Beans (page 142)
> Watermelon
> Coconut Cream Pielettes (page 219)

Not every lunch needs to go to work or school—have some fun! Pack a basket with tasty sandwiches and go to the park on a beautiful summer day. **Baked beans** and creamy **potato salad** make excellent picnic and potluck fare, especially when the potato salad is made with no mayonnaise.

POST-THANKSGIVING LUNCH BOX

My Favorite Tofurky Sandwich (page 88)
Mixed green salad with dried cranberries
    and almond slices
Caramelized Squash and Apples (page 163)
Glorified Rice (page 222)

Thanksgiving traditionally involves a whole roast turkey placed prominently at the center of an enormous feast. Happily, in the last few years another tradition has been born: the famous Thanksgiving **Tofurky**! Tofurky Roasts come filled with savory stuffing and are an easy vegan turkey alternative that anyone can make. In fact, Tofurky is now a best-seller here in the United States. Although I generally prefer doing most of my cooking from scratch, I get a special kick out of preparing a Tofurky Roast for Thanksgiving. Our son even gets to carve it with an electric carving knife! To find out more about Tofurky, visit www.tofurky.com.

As many Americans know, the very best part of Thanksgiving is eating all the leftovers. Make a Tofurky Roast and the side dishes above and you'll have a fantastic, easy-to-assemble lunch the next day.

THE SOUTHWEST

Corncob Cornbread (page 189) wrapped in
   "cornhusks" (see below)
Anasazi Beans (page 139)
Baby Squash Medley (page 162)
Fried Nopales (page 167)
Prickly Pear Pudding (page 229)

This lunch showcases some of the traditional foods of the southwestern region of the United States, including Arizona, New Mexico, Utah, and Colorado. Many of these foods have been eaten by Native Americans in this region for centuries.

Wrapping "cornhusks" around the outside of a piece of corncob-shaped **cornbread** is a fanciful way to pack some tortillas for scooping up bites of beans and nopales in this lunch: use scissors to trim corn tortillas into oval cornhusk shapes. Lay some down in the bottom of your cornbread container, place the cornbread in the middle, then wrap extra corn husk tortillas around the outside, leaving a bit of the cornbread peeking out the top.

SPORTS ALL-STAR

Jennifer's Omega-3 Protein Bars (page 55)
A vegan hot dog
All-Star Corn (page 159)
Yellow and red watermelon slices
Beverage: Grape Sports Drink (page 235)

My son is in love with American football. It took him a few years to talk his mom into letting him play such a violent, full-contact sport. I mean, hello, they're crashing into each other out there! On purpose!

But like many, many American boys and girls, he absolutely loves it, and I'm glad he's found a sport that keeps him active and fit. This lunch is for James and all the other school athletes out there who love to rock it on the sports field.

2

CANADA

SPRINGTIME IN QUEBEC

Ployes (Buckwheat Crêpes) (page 191)
Maple syrup or Frugal Momma's
    "Maple" Syrup (page 60)
Vegan Canadian bacon
Steamed fiddleheads (see below) or asparagus spears
Dried blueberries and cranberries

I didn't know what to include in a Canadian-inspired lunch box until I spoke with my good friend Renee Pottle, fellow healthy chef and author of *Homestyle Favorites Made Meatless*. She hails from the tip of Maine and was able to steer me in the direction of **ployes**: buckwheat crêpes made throughout the St. John Valley, the Acadian Maritimes, and Quebec. Best of all, they're naturally vegan! Slice them or roll them into tubes, and pack them with a small container of maple syrup for dipping and a slice of **vegan Canadian bacon** (we like Yves brand) for a breakfast-style lunch.

Fiddleheads are the unfurled fronds of a young edible fern. Foraging for them is a favorite springtime activity in New England and eastern Canada. According to Renee, they have an earthy flavor. They should be cooked and eaten quickly after harvesting: rinse them well in several changes of water and steam them until tender. Substitute **asparagus** if you don't have fiddleheads where you live.

3

MEXICO

I covered a lot of ground in our love of Mexico food in my first book, *Vegan Lunch Box*; there you'll find recipes for tamales, tortilla wraps, layered bean dip, empanadas, and more. Here are just two more Mexican menus that are hard to resist.

MEXICO #1

Flautas (page 116)
Salsa for dipping
Mexican Fruit Salad (page 208)
Tossed green salad with salsa for dressing
Avocaditos (see below)

A *flauta*, or "flute," is a corn tortilla rolled around a savory filling (in this case, refried beans) and fried until golden and crispy. There was quite a debate on my blog about whether these should be called *flautas* or *taquitos*, as the dishes are quite similar and the terminology seems to differ by region. I've decided to stick with calling them flautas, with the understanding that flautas are a bit thicker and looser than the tightly wrapped taquitos.

What could be more perfect for a packed lunch than miniature avocados you don't need to peel or pit? **Avocaditos**, also called cocktail avocados, are tiny, 3-inch long seedless avocados with thin, edible skin. Pack one or two in your lunchbox and slice them into rounds to nibble on at lunchtime. Or, if you'd rather not eat the skin, wait until the avocaditos are fully ripe, then slice off one end and squeeze out the flesh.

If you can't find avocaditos, pack half of a regular full-size avocado, rubbed with lemon juice and wrapped tightly in plastic wrap to prevent discoloration. Slice or mash at lunchtime for a rich, creamy treat.

MEXICO #2

Nacho Cheese Dip (page 63)
Baked tortilla chips
Sugar snap peas and bell pepper strips
A whole wheat tortilla filled with refried beans
Fresh strawberries

Nachos were invented in the 1940s by an ingenious maitre d' in Piedras Negras, Mexico, near the border with Texas. When he couldn't find the chef one evening, the maitre d' grabbed tostadas, cheese, and jalapeños, and invented the nacho to feed his hungry customers.

Over the years the cheese topping has transformed into a melted cheese sauce, and nachos have become a popular fast-food snack throughout the United States. This vegan version is just as creamy and flavorful as the dairy-laden version, but it's all-natural and much healthier. I say it even tastes better! For lunch, pack the warm **nacho dip** in an insulated food jar and serve it with tortilla chips, vegetables, and tortillas for dipping.

CENTRAL AND SOUTH AMERICA

EL SALVADOR

Pupusas (page 129)
Tomato sauce
Curtido (page 181)
Fresh melon slices

El Salvador's most popular snack is the **pupusa**, a thick masa flatbread stuffed with beans, potatoes, or other savory fillings. The pupusas are topped with spicy tomato sauce and *curtido*, a cabbage salad with a hot hint of chile. Pack tomato sauce and curtido in separate containers and top the pupusas with the sauce at lunchtime.

ANCIENT INCAN INSPIRATION

Quinoa Veggies (page 151)
Perfect Pinto Beans (page 146)
Baby bananas
Beverage: Mexican Hot Chocolate (page 240)

The ancient Incan people lived in what is now Peru, in South America. The three pillars of the Incan diet were corn (maize), potatoes, and **quinoa**. Quinoa (pronounced "KEEN-wah") is a small, quick-cooking, gluten-free grain that the world is now rediscovering. Quinoa was so essential to the Incan people that is was revered as *la chisiya mama*, the "Mother Grain." And no wonder! Quinoa is a complete protein and a good source of iron, phosphorus, and magnesium.

This lunch ends with an ancient, sacred beverage: **hot chocolate!** The cacao tree, that great giver of chocolate, is native to South America, and thus the ancient peoples of South America were the first to consume it. They drank chocolate in a way that would be unfamiliar to us: mixed with water, unsweetened, and spiced with hot chile powder (don't worry—that's not the recipe we'll be using in this lunch!). It was Europeans who introduced chocolate to sugar—a marriage made in heaven.

THE CARIBBEAN

CARIBBEAN #1

Plantain Wraps with Tangy Black Bean Spread (page 89)
Salsa for dipping
Caribbean Coleslaw (page 78)

The Caribbean is a chain of hundreds of islands that run in a curve from Florida in the north to Venezuela in the south. The cooking there is influenced by the climate; tropical fruits, sugarcane, and spices grow there in abundance.

In this Caribbean-inspired menu, cooked plantains and black beans come together in a wrap sandwich. On the side is a **coleslaw**, also inspired by the islands: limes and pineapple sweeten the dish.

CARIBBEAN #2

Bahama Mama's Beans and Rice (page 105)
Trinidad Spinach (page 185)
Fresh guava (see below) or other tropical fruit

Coconut milk serves as a rich, flavorful cooking liquid for **beans and rice** in many parts of the Caribbean. Serve it with an Indian-inspired **spinach** dish from the island of Trinidad and some fresh tropical fruit for dessert.

If you can find fresh **guava** in your area, you're in for a treat. Guava are small round fruit about the size of small eggs; when ripe, you can cut them open and eat them with a spoon. They are sweet and fragrant, with a scent like strawberries, and their flesh ranges in color from yellow to orange to a stunning hot pink.

WESTERN EUROPE

ENGLAND

English Kidney (Bean) Pie or Shepherd's Pie (page 114)
Sweet Peas with Mint (page 182)
Sour Cream Scones (page 192)
Lady apples (see below)

In England, many meals traditionally focus on a main dish of meat served with potatoes, or wrapped in pastry crust for a savory pie. Here is a little pie with the traditional "beefy" flavor of an English Kidney Pie, but I've let the cows hold on to their kidneys and filled it with kidney beans instead. For dessert, I adore this old English tea-time favorite any time of day: fresh-baked scones studded with currants.

Lady apples are the oldest known variety of cultivated apple, grown throughout Europe for centuries. Lady apples are very, very small apples—two or three bites and they're gone! Look for these tiny red and green wonders at grocery stores in the fall.

FRANCE

Ratatouille (page 101)
New potatoes or baguette bread
Comice pears
A bar of vegan dark chocolate

Ratatouille! Your kids love the movie, but have they tried the dish? Make this famous French country stew at the end of summer when eggplants, tomatoes, zucchini, and peppers are producing at breakneck speed. Serve Ratatouille over boiled, sliced new potatoes for a hearty gluten-free meal, or with slices of crusty **baguette bread** on the side. **Comice pears**—fat, green pears with a rosy blush, first grown in France in the 1800s—and a bar of **vegan dark chocolate** are *magnifique* for dessert.

A CHILD'S LUNCH IN FRANCE

Nancy Rigal, a researcher and senior lecturer on developmental child psychology at the University of Paris at Nanterre, has written a fascinating book on why children eat the way they do, entitled *Winning the Food Fight: How to Introduce Variety into Your Child's Diet.*

Reading descriptions of Rigal's studies made me acutely aware of the vast difference between the food culture of France and the one here in the United States. In one French study of 2- to 3-year-old children eating lunch at a day care, cauliflower "was chosen in 51% of the cases when prepared au gratin, in 49% when served with a béchamel sauce." Tomatoes were chosen in 52% of the cases when stuffed, but only 27% when served "à la Provençale."

Wow. Where I live, 2- to 3-year-olds in day care don't usually get a chance to choose cauliflower or tomatoes in any style, shape, or form. It's generally more of a choice between dinosaur-shaped meat nuggets or ones shaped like stars.

GERMANY

Cabbage Rolls (page 108)
Beet Salad (page 76)
Applesauce (page 205)
Spitzbuben (Little Rascals) (page 232)

Delicious **Cabbage Rolls** filled with a vegan "meatloaf" and baked in tomato sauce make an exciting lunch or a great main dish for potlucks and holiday celebrations. Homemade **Beet Salad**, **Applesauce**, and jam-filled sandwich cookies add more German flavor to this meal.

QUICK AND EASY VARIATION: There are two shortcuts you can take to make this menu easier: substitute store-bought applesauce for homemade, and canned pickled beets for the Beet Salad.

ITALY #1

Grilled Vegetable Stromboli (page 193)
Pesto or marinara sauce for dipping
Mixed green salad with Italian dressing
Balsamic Strawberries (page 206)

Bake this handsome Italian sandwich for your next packed lunch, family picnic, or game night with friends. **Stromboli** is shaped and baked with the filling rolled into it—in this case a mix of grilled vegetables and roasted garlic. When it's cool, cut the loaf into thick slices to share, with pesto or marina on the side for dipping.

For dessert, celebrate another delicacy from Italy—balsamic vinegar—by showcasing it on a bowl of fresh, sweet strawberries. It may seem unusual, but you'll find that balsamic syrup makes sweet strawberries taste even sweeter.

ITALY #2

Caponata Sandwiches (page 86)
Tri-colored pasta spirals tossed with olive oil
Mini Vegan Cheesecakes (page 226)
Mixed berries

Caponata is a sweet-and-sour eggplant relish, wonderful when sandwiched between slices of crusty Italian bread. Pack with a simple side of cooked **pasta spirals** and a muffin-size **vegan cheesecake** topped with **fresh berries**.

SCOTLAND

Vegetarian haggis (see below) or vegan sausages
Colcannon (page 164)
Brambles and berries (see below)
Brown Sugar Shortbread (page 215)

In Scotland, **haggis** is the centerpiece dish at the traditional Burns Night Dinner honoring Scotland's national poet, Robert Burns. The dish is presented with much ceremony along with the recitation of Burns's poem "Address to a Haggis." One would imagine that any recipe that starts out calling for the heart, lungs, and liver of a sheep would not be a good candidate for veganizing. But you would be wrong! Several brands of vegan haggis are on the market, including Celtic Croft ("made from the innards of the Highland soy-beast o' course"!), Macsweens, and Stahly Quality Foods. If haggis isn't of interest to you, substitute some fried vegan sausages.

Blackberries are known as **brambles** in Scotland, and they often grow wild in the hedgerows there. Other soft berries enjoyed in

Scotland include raspberries, strawberries, blackcurrant, redcurrant, whitecurrant, and gooseberries. Include a mix of colorful berries in your lunch for a cheerful, healthy treat.

SPAIN

Espinacas con Garbanzos
   (Spinach with Chickpeas) (page 165)
Sliced artisan bread
Patatas Bravas (Fierce Potatoes) (page 172)
Banderillas (page 68)
Grapes and orange slices

Enjoy a trio of classic *tapas*—Spanish appetizers served in bars all over Spain—in your lunch box. It is a fine Spanish tradition to stroll from tapas bar to tapas bar in the evening with friends, enjoying numerous "little bites" as you go. The three dishes here—flavorful **spinach cooked with chickpeas**, **"fierce" potatoes** in hot tomato sauce, and **Banderillas**—a selection of pickles and olives—make an enjoyable noontime meal, especially when packed along with a wedge of crusty **artisan-style bread** and some fresh fruit for dessert.

CENTRAL AND EASTERN EUROPE

HUNGARY

Hungary is known for hearty, filling dishes like traditional sour cream–rich Chicken Paprikás (pronounced "pah-pree-COSH"). This satisfying vegan version wouldn't be complete without some type of noodle or dumpling, so I serve it with a pretty side dish of noodles tossed with poppy seeds.

Kohlrabi is much loved in Eastern Europe but sadly underappreciated here in the West. This little member of the brassica family tastes like tender broccoli stalks. It looks strange but is simple to prepare: use a sharp paring knife to pare away the skin and stalks. The flesh near the root can be tough, so cut away the base of the bulb near the root, including any flesh that seems especially hard or stringy. Dice the rest of the flesh and steam until tender, about 8 to 10 minutes. Add a few frozen peas toward the end of cooking time.

RUSSIA

Kasha Kupecheskaya (page 122)
Heavenly Mushrooms (page 168)
Mixed greens salad
Russian Tea Cakes (page 231)
Pear slices

An old Russian proverb says, "You can't feed a Russian without kasha." Here is **kasha**—cooked toasted buckwheat kernels—with golden caramelized onions, enough to feed a hearty Russian appetite or your own. Tofu takes the place of the traditional hard-boiled egg.

I would add to that old saying that you also can't feed a Russian without **mushrooms**. The best mushrooms I've ever eaten were prepared for me by a Russian immigrant friend, who told me how they would hunt for wild mushrooms in her native country, and how mushrooms were considered an important meat replacer during the Orthodox fasts.

CHAPTER

8

THE MIDDLE EAST

ISRAEL

Mini Pita Bread (page 198)
Hummus
Baked Falafel (page 141)
Cucumber Tomato Salad (page 80)
Fresh pomegranate seeds

Falafel—round balls made from ground chickpeas and spices—are served all over the Middle East and are especially popular in Israel. For this lunch I've included homemade **Mini Pita Breads**; fill them with your favorite **hummus**, some lettuce or baby spinach, and some sprouts. Pack the Baked Falafel on the side to eat as finger food, or tuck them right into the pita.

LEBANON

Mujaddara (page 128)
Roasted Veggie Kabobs (page 178)
Stuffed Dates (page 212)
Beverage: Peach Smoothie (page 241)

Mujaddara is another dish that is served widely throughout the Middle East. It has been thought of as a food for the poor because the humble ingredients—rice, lentils, and onions—are cheap and easy to obtain. In this case, however, the poor have it best, as the flavors in this dish are beyond compare.

MOROCCO

Moroccan Tagine (page 97)
Orange Couscous (page 150)
Cinnamon-Sugar Almonds (page 151)
Tangerine slices

Although Morocco is in North Africa, it is part of the Middle Eastern cultural area, having more in common culturally and food-wise with the Middle East than with the rest of Africa.

A **tagine** is a thick Moroccan stew studded with chickpeas, vegetables, and raisins and served on a bed of couscous. A tagine is traditionally made in—what else?—a tagine, a special earthenware dish with a distinctive conical lid. I've kept it simple and made this version in a regular saucepan. **Cinnamon-Sugar Almonds** and fresh **tangerines** (named after the city of Tangier, in Morocco!) make a captivating Moroccan-inspired dessert.

TURKEY

Stuffed Eggplants (page 131)
Fresh Fava Bean Salad (page 143)
Mini Pita Bread (page 198)
Turkish Delight (see below)

This is a stunning lunch, combining the beauty and flavor of **stuffed baby eggplants** with the vivid green of a **Fresh Fava Bean Salad**. (I don't think there's anything quite as green as a fresh fava bean.) Homemade **pita breads** stand ready to scoop up salad and eggplant alike.

Turkish Delight (*lokum*) is a soft jellied candy made from vegan ingredients, mainly water, sugar, cornstarch, and cream of tartar. Nuts like pistachios or walnuts, rosewater, and citrus are common flavorings. If you have a hard time finding authentic Turkish Delight in your area, the familiar American-made candy "Aplets and Cotlets" (made right here in my own state of Washington) is available in grocery stores or online at www.aplets.com.

INDIA

Mung Dahl (page 144)
Steamed basmati rice
Palak Paneer (page 171)
Naan (Indian Flatbread) (page 200)
Fresh mango

If anyone you know is still doubtful that people can survive and thrive on a vegetarian diet, point them to India. Millions of people in India live their entire lives as vegetarians, in the same land where generations of their ancestors were also vegetarian. Hindus, Buddhists, and Jains in India follow the precept of *ahimsa*, or nonviolence, and abstain from killing animals for food. They have spent thousands of years perfecting this cuisine, and it shows in the complexity of tastes, textures, and flavors in their amazing dishes, a small part of which this menu is intended to capture.

LUNCH IN MUMBAI

If you were going to work or school in Mumbai, India, you might not have to carry your own lunch. Your stacked metal tiffin (lunch box) would be picked up at your home and delivered to you promptly at lunchtime by a "tiffinwalla" (lunch deliverer), who would then retrieve your empty tiffin and return it to your home to be filled again the next day. Amazingly, tiffinwallas in Mumbai deliver over 175,000 lunches like this every day!

AFRICA

Africa is an enormous continent. People in the Western world tend to think of Africa as one place, one culture. But Africa is home to an enormous array of regional cultures and cuisines. Instead of trying to do justice to each of them in one small book, I chose instead to create two menus representing some of the ingredients that are widely used in many areas around the continent, such as black-eyed peas, plantains, and greens.

If you are interested in African cuisine, be sure not to miss the Ethiopian recipes in my first cookbook, *Vegan Lunch Box.*

AFRICA #1

Black-Eyed Peas and Potatoes with
   Cilantro and Lime (page 107)
Oven Roasted Okra (page 170)
Plantain Chips (page 57)
Honeydew melon

Tender **black-eyed peas** and other cowpeas (also called "crowder peas" here in the United States, because they're all crowded together in their pods) are served all over the African continent. Like all legumes and pulses, they're a great source of protein. Add some whole roasted **okra** on the side—another nutritious vegetable from Africa.

Fried **plantain chips** make an interesting, African-inspired snack; they taste like a cross between potato chips and dried banana chips. Plantains are very popular in West Africa and the Caribbean. They may look like giant bananas, but watch out! Although they're members of the banana family, they aren't sweet and shouldn't be eaten raw.

A sad little monkey sings about his accidental purchase of plantains at Rathergood (http://www.rathergood.com/bananas/). Too bad he didn't know about plantain chips!

AFRICA #2

Jollof Rice (page 120)
African Greens (page 157)
A baby banana

Many variations of **Jollof Rice** are served throughout West Africa. The dish is a spicy mixture of rice, meat (in this case, chicken-style seitan), vegetables, tomatoes, and onions. It's a delicious meal all by itself, but even better teamed up here with some creamy **African Greens**.

Bananas are ubiquitous throughout Africa, and a baby banana or two will fit perfectly in this or any lunch box. I once packed lunch for some young members of the African Children's Choir. They were delighted with the baby bananas and told me they were "like the bananas in Uganda." Remember, it's easiest to open them from the bottom, not the top.

CHAPTER

11

ASIA

CHINA

Tofu Char Sui (page 132)
Teriyaki Green Beans (page 184)
Short-grain rice
Steamed dumplings (see below)
Mandarin oranges and kiwifruit
   (also known as Chinese gooseberries!)

I created this Chinese menu on Chinese New Year during my son's first year at school and tucked in a little note talking about the "Year of the Dog" and what it meant. In the rush of school lunches that followed afterward, I promptly forgot about it.

At the end of the school year I decided it would be fun to do a "Top Ten" countdown on the Vegan Lunch Box blog. I asked James what his favorite lunches of the year had been, expecting to hear a list of veggie dogs, potato chips, and cookies.

He didn't hesitate for a moment. "Chinese!" he said.

"Chinese?" I asked, completely confused. "What lunch was that?"

"You know, it had teriyaki green beans, and a dumpling, and that tofu. That was my favorite!"

I almost fell over in astonishment. It had been such an out-of-the-ordinary lunch, and he hadn't mentioned it since the day he ate it. But apparently it had made a strong—and positive—impression on him.

We all expect our children to want nothing but bland "kid food" and sugary sweets, but here is a well-balanced lunch filled with vegetables, fresh fruit, and vegan protein . . . and it turns out to be a first grader's all-time favorite!

Look for heavenly **steamed dumplings** in the freezer at your local Asian market. They are white in color and look like smooth, round balls. The outside of the dumpling is made from wheat dough; the inside can hold any number of fillings. Most fillings are made with meat or seafood; look for vegetable dumplings or dumplings filled with sweet bean paste (those are our favorites). Here's how to prepare them once you get them home: place each dumpling on a square of parchment or wax paper brushed with a bit of vegetable oil. Place the dumplings in a steamer basket over boiling water. Make sure the dumplings do not touch each other or the sides of the steamer, or they will stick. Steam until heated through, about 10 minutes.

KOREA

Rice with Toasted Millet (page 153)
Kimchi (see below)
Bean Sprout Salad (page 75)
Stir-Fried Watercress (page 181)
Vegan meatballs with Korean Dipping Sauce (page 61)
Fresh plums

Traditional Korean meals feature a wide assortment of *panchan*, or side dishes, surrounding a main dish of rice or noodles. Diners pick and choose from the many *panchan*, adding a bit of something spicy to one bite of rice, a bit of something crunchy to the next, and so on.

One of these side dishes is always, of course, the Korean national food **kimchi**. Kimchi is a brine-fermented vegetable, usually cabbage. There are countless varieties of kimchi, ranging from mild to super-hot spicy. Look for kimchi at Asian markets and in the produce section at some grocery stores. Double-check to ensure that the one you choose is vegan; some kimchi contains fish or shrimp paste.

Along with the vegetables and rice in this healthy lunch, I've included a serving of **vegan meatballs**. Look for packaged vegan meatballs in the freezer section at your local grocery or health food store (I highly recommend "Nate's Meatless"). Bake the meatballs according to package directions and pack with a decorative food pick and a container of **Korean Dipping Sauce**.

INDONESIA

Golden Indonesian Tempeh (page 117)
Yellow Coconut Rice (page 156)
Indonesian Vegetable Pickles (page 169)
Tangerine or orange slices and star fruit (carambola)
Beverage: Iced Lemongrass Tisane (page 237)

Indonesia: land of **tempeh**! I absolutely *adore* tempeh. It's got a nutty, mushroomy flavor and a very impressive nutritional profile. For those who haven't met tempeh yet, it is made from cooking and fermenting whole soybeans until they form solid cakes that can be cut into slices and steamed or fried. It's got more bioavailable protein than tofu or plain cooked soybeans, and the fermentation of tempeh makes it easier to digest. Thank you, Indonesia!

THAILAND #1

Pad Thai (see below)
Red Curry Vegetables (page 176)
Thai Cucumber Salad (page 84)
An Asian Pear

Pad Thai has finally gone vegan! Pad Thai—"Thai style" stir-fried rice noodles—typically contain fish sauce, one of the essential flavors in Thai cooking. But now, several prepackaged Pad Thai mixes that don't contain fish are available in the Asian section at grocery stores. A Taste of Thai "Pad Thai for Two" is our favorite. For a quick and easy meal, follow the directions on the package, substituting slices of firm tofu for the meat and leaving out the egg. Garnish with mung bean sprouts, chopped peanuts if you like, and a wedge of lime.

Asian Pears were once grown primarily in Asia but have become increasingly popular in the United States. It's no wonder why: Asian Pears combine the crisp crunch of an apple with the flavor of a sweet, juicy pear. In fact, they have also been called "apple pears"! Asian Pears look like yellow or light green apples and have white flesh. Look for them in most grocery stores.

THAILAND #2

Mango Noodles (page 124)
Basil Salad with Lime and Red Curry Dressing (page 38)
Beverage: Thai Iced Tea (page 242)

Here's another stir-fried rice noodle dish, this one made from scratch. If you've never worked with rice noodles before, you'll find them fast and easy; a brief soak in hot water and they are ready to go.

THE PAD THAI DISASTER,
OR "NEVER SAY NEVER"

My son has always been an adventurous eater, willing and eager to try everything at least once. The first time James tried Pad Thai was when he was four years old, at a cozy little Thai restaurant. He had been happily munching on tofu satay (plain grilled tofu on a stick: one of the most picky-kid-friendly dishes at a Thai restaurant) when he asked if he could try one of the rice noodles from his father's plate. He placed the noodle in his mouth, chewed once, and promptly threw up all over the table. I was mortified beyond my wildest nightmares. I rushed him off to the bathroom while the waitress earned possibly the largest tip ever by clearing off the table. I thought right then and there that rice noodles were out forever. Never, never, never again would my son be given a rice noodle.

But four years later, when James was eight, he grabbed one of the Pad Thai boxes off the shelf at the grocery store and asked if he could give it a try. I paled at the mere thought of it. With no small amount of trepidation, I bought the package and took it home. At dinner, I put some noodles on his plate and ran for cover.

Lo and behold, he loved it! Pad Thai is now one of his favorite Thai dishes, and he eats it with gusto. Watching him inhaling rice noodles always reminds me that tastes can change, and that it's never too late to learn to like something that you didn't care for (or positively gagged on) the first time.

VIETNAM

Vegetarian Pho (page 103)
Vietnamese Salad Rolls (page 91)
Hoisin sauce for dipping
Fresh or drained canned lychee fruit (see below)

Pho (pronounced something like "fuh") is a staple of Vietnamese cuisine, a flavorful soup eaten for breakfast, lunch, or dinner. The soup is traditionally served with a variety of fresh ingredients to add in just before you take each bite, such as scallions, cilantro, basil, and wedges of lime. Enjoy your Pho alongside a **Vietnamese Salad Roll** filled with crunchy lettuce and Asian-flavored portobello mushrooms.

Fresh **lychee fruit** are quite a treat if you can find them. They are tiny fruits covered in rough red skin that is easily peeled away to reveal the sweet, translucent fruit. Eat the fruit away from the center seed and discard the seed. If you can't find fresh, lychee are also good canned.

VEGETARIAN IN VIETNAM

" . . . Vegetarianism is a form of merit-making. In Asian culture, it's not uncommon for one to abstain from eating meat as a way to *duoc phuoc* (gain merit). In doing so, one's wishes would be granted."

—Mai Pham, *Pleasures of the Vietnamese Table*

AUSTRALIA

LUNCH DOWN UNDER

Vegemite Sandwich (page 90)
Baked crisps (baked potato chips)
Paw-paw (papaya)
Lamingtons (page 224)

Vegemite is so popular in Australia (nine out of ten Australia kitchens contain it) it's become a symbol of the nation. Just like American children fall back on peanut butter and jelly for a quick lunch or snack, Australian children reach for the Vegemite.

I couldn't resist including a serving of **fresh papaya** in this lunch menu, a fruit known as **paw-paw** in the north of Australia (not to be confused with the native American fruit also called paw-paw or prairie banana). My grandmother grew up near her uncle's paw-paw farm in Queensland and told stories of plucking them ripe from the trees and eating them in the shade. She missed them after she moved to the United States; back then fresh papaya was something you could only dream about in the deserts of eastern Washington.

For dessert, **Lamingtons** are another classic Australian treat: sweet cubes of sponge cake dipped in chocolate and rolled in coconut.

A CHILD'S LUNCH IN AUSTRALIA

I recently asked family friend Casey Bell, an early childhood teacher in Australia, what schoolchildren in Australia eat for lunch:

Australian kids' lunches are very dependent on seasons. In most of Australia children live through four seasons (summer, autumn, winter, spring) so their lunch box contents depend on what is available at the time. In summer we eat cherries, peaches, plums, nectarines, grapes, and bananas, and in winter we eat oranges and apples. In the north of the country the children eat more tropical fruits such as mango and paw-paw.

In the north of the country (Darwin, Cairns, etc.) there are only two seasons: the wet season (hot with rain) and the dry season (hot without rain). So in these schools there are generally fridges in each classroom. However, in my experience they generally eat sandwiches, fruit, packaged things like muesli bars, etc. In most schools there is a ban on anything that can cause severe allergies, such as eggs and peanut butter.

"We encourage our kids to drink lots of water, especially in the summer time. Our school canteens are going through huge overhauls to concentrate on more healthy, fresh, and nutritious foods.

CHAPTER 13

JAPAN

Now here we are at last in the land that is my biggest inspiration: **Japan**, the country where packing lunch has become a minor art form.

"Bento moms" (and dads!) across Japan practice the fine art of bento every day. Their lunches are expertly composed, well-balanced, and beautiful to look at. The real pros even make bento lunches into miniature portraits of their child's favorite things, like dinosaurs, rocket ships, princesses, video game scenes, or anime cartoon characters. Although they look too pretty to eat, nothing is left of them by the late afternoon!

HOW TO PACK LUNCH LIKE A BENTO SUPERSTAR

- Pick out a bento box or other compact lunch container that will hold your food with no room left over; bento boxes are packed snugly so there is no shifting of contents or wasted space.
- Pack the largest section of your bento with a filling carbohydrate such as rice, sushi rolls, or noodles. The main dish (for example, a

serving of stir-fried vegetables with tofu) should go alongside the rice and take up less than half the space. It's also common to include small servings of several dishes instead of one main dish; try to balance the flavors, textures, and colors, and include two to four bites of each.

- If you do end up with extra space inside your box, fill it in with small items like cherry tomatoes, lettuce leaves, edamame, strawberries, broccoli florets, or a piece of candy.

- Add playful garnishes—little touches to make your bento beautiful. For example, it's common to use paper punches to make "happy faces" from sheets of nori seaweed. Place them on top of *onigiri* (rice balls), sandwiches, vegetables, or tofu. Other pretty garnishes include small hearts, flowers, or stars cut from vegetables like carrot or daikon. You can also use cookie cutters to cut fruits like melon or kiwifruit into decorative shapes.

- Use bento accessories. Colorful plastic dividers can keep your foods from touching each other. Plastic or paper food cups (or regular cupcake liners turned inside-out) can hold small servings of food. Squeeze bottles for things like soy sauce and salad dressing come in fun shapes like fish, pigs, flowers, and teddy bears. Add decorative food picks or tiny forks to eat fruit and other small nibbles. Accessories like these and more are available online at Web sites such as I Love Obento (www.iloveobento.com).

JAPAN #1: TAMAGOYAKI BENTO

Tofu Tamagoyaki (page 133)
Potato Salad Balls (page 58)
Cucumber Sushi Rolls (page 52)
Octo-Celery (page 71)
Kiwifruit and watermelon
Botan Rice Candy (see below)

Here's a nice example of a well-rounded bento lunch, with a pleasantly diverse assortment of colors, tastes, and textures to choose from. Pack two or three of each item, arranging them attractively and filling any leftover space with small bits of lettuce or cherry tomatoes.

Botan Rice Candy are chewy candies wrapped in an edible layer of rice paper. Put them in your mouth and the paper dissolves. Botan Rice Candy is available in the Asian section of grocery stores or at Asian markets.

JAPAN #2: ONIGIRI BENTO

Onigiri (rice balls) (page 148)
Vegan chicken nuggets
Stir-Fried Arame with Carrots and Ginger (page 179)
Radish Rosettes (page 72)
Apple Bunnies (page 203)

Another classic bento. This one features one of the most common lunch box items in Japan: **onigiri**. Onigiri are simple rice balls, shaped by hand or with a mold, that can be picked up and eaten by hand. Sheets of nori are used like edible paper to decorate the outside of the onigiri.

JAPAN #3: ZARU SOBA BENTO

Zaru Soba (page 136)
Edamame
Carrot and Daikon Salad (page 79)
Fuyu persimmon (see below)

Zaru Soba was another surprise hit during my son's first year at school; he even included this menu in his list of "Top Ten" at the end of the year. Zaru Soba are cold buckwheat noodles, picked up with chopsticks and dipped into a flavorful broth just before eating.

Persimmons, or *kaki*, are grown and eaten widely in Japan. Fuyu persimmons are squat, reddish-orange fruit that resemble tomatoes. Fuyus are firm when ripe and taste something like a spiced apple (don't confuse the squat Fuyu with the heart-shaped Hachiya, which is very soft when ripe and must be eaten with a spoon). Slice them into rounds or wedges and pack them in the lunch box with a decorative food pick.

JAPAN #4: TIGER BENTO

Tofu Tiger (page 134)
Japanese short-grain rice
Carrot-Cucumber Tulips (page 69)
Broccoli Salad with Daikon Flowers (page 77)
Strawberries

After posting a picture of this lunch on my blog, one of my readers reported that her son was so delighted by it that she ordered him his very own Laptop Lunch Box. When the box arrived he excitedly rushed to open it, and then his face fell. "Where's the tiger?" he asked.

Part 2
THE RECIPES

APPETIZERS AND SNACKS

BARLEY CRACKERS

These pretty little crackers are studded with poppy seeds. Cut them out in any shape you like, adjusting the baking time upward for larger crackers.

Makes several dozen small crackers

½ cup canola oil

2 cups all-purpose flour

1 cup barley flour

½ teaspoon baking soda

½ teaspoon kosher salt

1 teaspoon poppy seeds

1 tablespoon apple cider vinegar

Olive oil

Salt, to taste

▶ Chill the canola oil in the freezer for at least 30 minutes before you begin, to allow it to thicken.

- Preheat the oven to 375°F. Line a baking sheet with parchment paper and set aside.
- In a medium mixing bowl, combine the flour, barley flour, baking soda, salt, and poppy seeds and whisk to combine. Drizzle in the canola oil and toss with your fingers until the oil is incorporated and the flour has formed small to medium-size clumps.
- Mix ½ cup ice water with the vinegar and drizzle it into the flour, stirring with your fingers until the dough holds together.
- Turn the dough out onto a lightly floured surface and knead just enough to form a cohesive dough. Divide the dough into three pieces, covering two with plastic as your roll out the first one.
- Lightly flour your work surface and roll the dough ⅛ inch thick. Cut out crackers using cookie cutters or a sharp knife and place them on the prepared baking sheet.
- Brush or spray the crackers lightly with olive oil and sprinkle with salt, if you like. Bake until golden, about 12 minutes.

Allergen Information ✳ Soy-free, nut-free. Contains gluten and wheat.

CINNAMON-SUGAR ALMONDS

Roasted nuts with a touch of sweet and a touch of salty are all the rage nowadays. It's easy and fun to make your own. Add a sprinkle of cayenne if you like your nuts sweet, salty, *and* spicy.

I prefer to use blanched whole almonds (whole almonds with the skins removed) for this recipe, but skin-on almonds are less expensive and easier to find.

Makes 1 cup

----
1 cup whole almonds, blanched or skin-on

1 teaspoon canola oil

1½ tablespoons sugar mixed with

　　¼ teaspoon cinnamon

⅛ teaspoon kosher salt

▸ Preheat the oven to 300°F. Spread the almonds out in a single layer on an ungreased baking sheet. Roast for 20 to 25 minutes, until fragrant and toasty. Shake the pan or stir the nuts with a wooden spoon occasionally so they roast evenly.

▸ Heat the canola oil in a saucepan or cast-iron skillet. Add the nuts and stir to coat with the oil. Add the cinnamon-sugar mixture and the salt. Cook, stirring constantly, until the sugar melts and starts to caramelize, about 5 minutes.

▸ Spread the nuts out on a plate to cool, stirring occasionally to keep them from sticking.

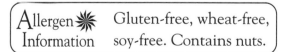

Allergen Information ✳ Gluten-free, wheat-free, soy-free. Contains nuts.

CUCUMBER SUSHI ROLLS

An easy alternative to regular sushi rolls. These little cucumber shells filled with rice make a cute snack or addition to any lunch box.

Makes 4 rolls

Special equipment you will need:
2 small graduated round cookie cutters

1 medium cucumber
1 cup prepared Sushi Rice (page 154)
Pickled ginger for serving (optional)
Soy sauce for serving

▸ Cut the cucumber into 1¼-inch rounds (use the container you plan to pack them in as a guide to make sure they will fit, making them smaller if necessary).

▸ Use a small (about 1-inch) round cookie cutter or apple corer to remove the core of the cucumber. Place the round on a hard surface and pack the center firmly with sushi rice.

▸ Now use a larger circular cookie cutter to cut away the peel and part of the flesh from the outside of the cucumber (about 1¼ to 1½ inch).

▸ Top the Sushi Rolls with pickled ginger, if desired, and serve with soy sauce for dipping.

Allergen ✳ Information   Gluten-free, wheat-free, soy-free, nut-free.

FISH CRACKERS

In some toddler circles Goldfish Crackers are like one of the four major food groups. Now vegan kids and those with dairy allergies can enjoy them, too! Nutritional yeast adds a hint of "cheesiness" and spices add extra flavor. But how can we make the crackers orange without cheddar? Well, surprisingly enough, cheese isn't what makes cheese crackers orange. It's actually natural annatto food coloring that does the trick. Annatto seed extract is used to color cheddar cheese and many other foods; of course, you can use any orange food coloring you wish or leave out the coloring for crackers that are wheat-colored but just as tasty. Before you begin, you'll need to purchase a tiny fish-shaped cookie cutter like the one available at www.coppergifts.com.

Makes several dozen crackers

½ cup canola oil

1¼ cups whole spelt flour

1½ cups all-purpose flour

4 tablespoons nutritional yeast flakes

¾ teaspoon baking soda

½ teaspoon salt

1 teaspoon paprika

⅛ teaspoon cayenne

½ teaspoon onion powder

¼ teaspoon garlic powder

½ cup ice water

1 tablespoon apple cider vinegar

Orange food coloring, as desired

Olive oil cooking spray

Fine sea salt, to taste

- Chill the canola oil in the freezer for at least 30 minutes before you begin, to allow it to thicken.
- Preheat the oven to 375°F. Line baking sheets with parchment paper and spray with nonstick spray.
- Combine the flours, nutritional yeast, baking soda, salt, paprika, cayenne, and onion and garlic powder in a medium mixing bowl and whisk to combine.
- Drizzle in the cold canola oil and toss with your fingers until the oil is incorporated and the flour has formed small to medium-size clumps.
- Mix the ice water and vinegar together.
- Add orange food coloring to the ice water mixture if desired. Drizzle the liquid over the flour, stirring with your fingers until the dough holds together.
- Turn out the dough onto a lightly floured work surface. Knead a few times, adding a bit more water if needed to form a cohesive dough. Use a rolling pin to roll the dough out thinly, about ⅛ inch thick.
- Cut out fish shapes using a small cookie cutter. If you would like to make happy fishies, use the curved tip of a spoon to give them a smile and a toothpick to give them an eye.
- Place the fish on the baking sheets, spray with olive oil and sprinkle with fine sea salt. Bake for 10 minutes, or until lightly golden on the bottom.
- Slide the parchment paper covered with fish onto a wire rack to cool.
- Continue rolling, cutting, and baking little fish until you just can't take it anymore.

Allergen ✳ Information — Soy-free, nut-free. Contains wheat and gluten.

JENNIFER'S OMEGA-3 PROTEIN BARS

I created these bars one summer when I was competing in a gym competition. I wanted a homemade alternative to expensive, pre-packaged protein bars and was also looking for a portable way to get my daily serving of omega-3 fatty acids from flaxseed. These bars were just the thing, rich in vegan protein and healthy fats, simple to make, and easy to tuck into a gym bag for an after-workout snack.

Makes 8 bars

½ cup quinoa flour

½ cup brown rice protein powder

1 cup ground flaxseed

½ teaspoon cinnamon

½ cup brown rice syrup

½ cup applesauce

¼ cup nut butter

½ cup raisins or other dried fruit

½ cup chopped walnuts

▸ Preheat oven to 350°F. Spray an 8 x 8-inch pan with nonstick spray and set aside.

▸ Mix the quinoa flour, protein powder, ground flaxseed, and cinnamon in a large mixing bowl. In another bowl combine the brown rice syrup, applesauce, and nut butter. Add the wet ingredients to the dry ingredients along with the raisins and walnuts.

▸ Knead the mixture together to form a soft dough (add a bit more flour if necessary to form a cohesive dough). Press the dough firmly and evenly into the prepared pan.

▸ Bake for 20 minutes, until the dough is partially cooked and holds together. Cut the dough into eight bars with a sharp knife and carefully lift each bar out with a spatula, pressing them into shape and placing them 1 inch apart on a baking sheet. Bake for 15 minutes, turn the bars over, and bake for another 15 minutes, or until the bars are nicely browned on both sides.

▸ Cool the bars on a wire rack and store in an airtight container in the refrigerator.

Allergen ✳ Information | Gluten-free, wheat-free, soy-free. Contains nuts.

PLANTAIN CHIPS

(Africa)

Plantains get sweeter as they turn progressively yellow then brown.
Use greener plantains for these chips.

Makes 4 servings

Canola or other oil for frying

2 green plantains

½ lemon

Salt, to taste

▸ Fill a saucepan or deep fryer with enough oil to submerge the chips (1½ to 2 inches or so). Heat the oil to 350°F (you will see the oil swirling and moving in the pot when it is hot enough). Adjust the heat as needed to maintain proper temperature; don't let the oil get too hot and start to smoke.

▸ Peel the plantains (using a paring knife helps) and rub them with the lemon to keep them from turning brown.

▸ Use a sharp knife or mandoline to cut the plantains into thin slices like potato chips.

▸ Fry the plantain chips in small batches, stirring them frequently with a slotted metal spoon to keep them from clumping. Fry until chips are golden yellow, about 1 minute.

▸ Transfer the plantain chips to a baking sheet lined with paper towels and sprinkle them with salt while they are still hot.

QUICK AND EASY VARIATION: If you don't feel like whipping out the Fry Daddy, ready-made plantain chips can be purchased at some specialty grocery stores or online at www.grabemsnacks.com

Allergen ✳ Information   Gluten-free, wheat-free, soy-free, nut-free.

POTATO SALAD BALLS

Kid Friendly

(Japan)

The first time I read about *jyagatama*—Japanese potato salad balls—I was skeptical. Could balls of mashed potato salad really taste good? I was wrong to have doubted the wisdom of the bento masters; these are not just good, they are addictive.

Makes 24 balls

3 large Yukon Gold potatoes, peeled and
    cut into ½-inch dice (about 4 cups)
⅓ to ½ cup mixed frozen vegetables, cooked
    according to package directions and drained
⅓ cup Vegenaise
1 tablespoon freshly squeezed lemon juice
¼ teaspoon sugar
Salt, to taste

▶ Bring a medium saucepan filled with salted water to a boil. Add the diced potatoes and cook until the potatoes are tender but not falling apart, about 12 minutes. Drain well.

▶ Place the drained potatoes in a large mixing bowl and gently mash them with a potato masher or wooden spoon. Don't keep mashing until the potatoes are smooth—there should still be lumps in the potatoes and the consistency should be coarse.

▶ Stir in the mixed vegetables, Vegenaise, lemon juice, sugar, and salt. Taste and adjust the seasoning as desired. When the mixture has cooled enough to handle, roll into 1-inch balls (measure your lunch container first—you may need to make the balls smaller to fit).

Allergen ✳ Information   Gluten-free, wheat-free, nut-free.
    Contains soy.

DIPS, SAUCES, AND SPREADS

CARAMEL DIP

This dip stays creamy and soft even when cold. Use it as a dip for apples, bananas, or winter pears.

Makes about 1½ cups	1 (8-ounce) container vegan cream cheese, softened ¾ cup packed brown sugar 1 teaspoon vanilla

▸ Blend all the ingredients together using a handheld mixer or a stand mixer fitted with the paddle attachment. Blend well for 2 minutes, until the sugar has dissolved. Refrigerate until needed.

Allergen Information ✳ Gluten-free, wheat-free, nut-free. Contains soy.

FRUGAL MOMMA'S "MAPLE" SYRUP

One of the things you may notice about vegan baking is the amount of maple syrup called for in many recipes. A lot of vegan cooks rely on maple syrup to take the place of honey and sugar in recipes, particularly in baked desserts. Sadly, with the price of real maple syrup going up and up, I just can't afford to use that much of it anymore. So, I devised this very simple, inexpensive recipe for homemade "maple" syrup using brown sugar and natural maple flavor. Look for bottles of maple flavor in the baking section of grocery and health food stores.

Makes 2 cups

2 cups firmly packed brown sugar

1 teaspoon cornstarch

1 cup water

1 teaspoon natural maple flavor

▸ Put the brown sugar into a medium saucepan. Put the cornstarch into a small bowl or cup and drizzle with about 2 tablespoons of the water. Stir or whisk with a fork until the cornstarch is dissolved, then add it to the saucepan along with the rest of the water. Stir or whisk constantly over medium-high heat until the mixture comes to a boil. Boil one minute, still stirring.

▸ Remove the saucepan from the heat and let the syrup cool completely. When it is cool, stir in the maple flavor. Store in the refrigerator.

Allergen ✳ Information   Gluten-free, wheat-free, soy-free, nut-free. Contains corn.

KOREAN DIPPING SAUCE

(Korea)

Serve this dipping sauce with vegan meatballs, fried tofu, or steamed or fried Asian dumplings.

Makes ⅓ cup
(1 to 2 servings)

1 tablespoon toasted sesame seeds

¼ cup low-sodium soy sauce

1 tablespoon rice vinegar

¼ teaspoon grated fresh ginger

¼ teaspoon Korean pepper powder
(*kochukaru*) or paprika (or, if you like it
spicy, use cayenne to taste)

Pinch of sugar

▶ Crush the sesame seeds lightly with a mortar and pestle. Combine the soy sauce, vinegar, ginger, pepper powder, and sugar in a small bowl and stir together. Stir in the sesame seeds.

Allergen ✳ Information — Gluten-free, wheat-free, nut-free. Contains soy.

MAUI ONION DIP

Slow roasting brings out the onions' natural sweetness in this amazing dip. Serve with fresh vegetable crudités or kettle chips.

Makes about
2 cups

2 large Maui onions (or other sweet onions,
    such as Vidalias or Walla Walla Sweets),
    peeled and quartered
1 tablespoon olive oil
⅓ cup vegan sour cream (I use Tofutti)
1 tablespoon freshly squeezed lemon juice
2 tablespoons fresh cilantro, roughly chopped
Pinch of cayenne (optional)
Salt and freshly ground black pepper, to taste

▸ Preheat oven to 400°F.

▸ Arrange the onions in a baking dish and drizzle with olive oil. Toss to coat and roast, stirring occasionally, until the onions are soft and golden, about 1 hour.

▸ Let the onions cool, then put them in a food processor fitted with the S blade along with the vegan sour cream, lemon juice, and cilantro. Pulse until blended but still chunky.

▸ Season with cayenne, salt, and pepper.

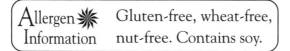 Allergen Information — Gluten-free, wheat-free, nut-free. Contains soy.

NACHO CHEESE DIP

My good friend Linda shared the original version of this fantastic recipe with me; we were all delighted by this creamy, cheesy nacho dip. Pour it on tortilla chips, tacos, and burritos or serve it as a warm dip with carrots, celery, and bell pepper strips.

Makes about
3 cups

2 cups water

¼ cup cooked white beans, drained

1 (4-ounce) jar pimentos or roasted red
    peppers, drained

1 cup nutritional yeast flakes

2 tablespoons cornstarch

1 tablespoon freshly squeezed lemon juice

1 teaspoon salt, or to taste

½ teaspoon onion powder

¼ teaspoon garlic powder

½ teaspoon cumin, heaping

¼ cup salsa or picante sauce

▸ Combine all ingredients in a blender and blend until completely smooth. Transfer the mixture to a medium saucepan and whisk constantly over medium heat until it comes to a boil. Simmer, whisking constantly, at least one minute or until thickened.

▸ Serve as a dip with tortilla chips and vegetables.

VARIATIONS: Add some Mexican-style vegetarian burger crumbles, black olives, diced chiles, or pickled jalapeños to the finished dip.

Allergen Information ☀ Gluten-free, wheat-free, soy-free, nut-free. Contains corn.

ROASTED GARLIC

Roasting works a positively magical transformation on the humble garlic head, transforming it into a collection of soft, spreadable cloves with a deep, mellow flavor. Warm roasted garlic makes a great spread for artisan-style bread or baguettes; squeeze the garlic from the clove directly onto a thick slice of bread and spread with a butter knife. Serve warm roasted heads of garlic as an appetizer at your next party, and save any leftovers to add to homemade bean spreads, mashed potatoes, or Grilled Vegetable Stromboli (page 193).

Makes 1 head of roasted garlic, easily increased

1 whole head of garlic

2 teaspoons olive oil

▸ Preheat the oven to 400°F.

▸ Use your hands to rub off most of the outer layers of skin from the garlic head, leaving the innermost layer surrounding the cloves intact.

▸ Use a sharp kitchen knife to cut the top ½ inch off the top of the head of garlic. This should cut the tips off the cloves and expose them at the top.

▸ Place the head of garlic on a square of aluminum foil. Drizzle the garlic with the olive oil and wrap up completely with the foil. Place the garlic bundle in a small baking pan or into the cup of a muffin pan.

▸ Roast for 30 minutes, until garlic is soft when pressed. Remove from foil and allow to cool slightly before using.

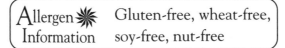

Allergen Information ✳ Gluten-free, wheat-free, soy-free, nut-free

ROASTED RED PEPPER SPREAD

This flavorful spread makes a nice, easy filling for celery sticks and tastes great in Baguette with Roasted Red Pepper Spread (page 85).

Makes about
2 cups

1 (7-ounce) jar roasted red peppers, drained
    well and finely chopped
1 (8-ounce) container vegan cream cheese,
    softened
3 tablespoons finely minced onion
1 small clove garlic, minced

▶ In a small mixing bowl combine the roasted red pepper, cream cheese, minced onion, and garlic. Chill until ready to use.

Allergen ✳ Information   Gluten-free, wheat-free, nut-free. Contains soy.

TANGY BLACK BEAN SPREAD

I like to use this zesty spread in sandwiches and wraps or as a dip for baby carrots.

Makes 4 to 6
servings

1 (15-ounce) can black beans, rinsed and
   drained
2 tablespoons freshly squeezed lemon juice
1½ tablespoons ketchup
2 teaspoons Bragg's Liquid Aminos or
   low-sodium soy sauce
½ teaspoon ground cumin
⅛ teaspoon cayenne, or to taste
Salt, to taste

▸ Blend all the ingredients together in a food processor fitted with the S blade, stopping to scrape down the sides once or twice. Blend until smooth. Taste and season with salt if desired.

Allergen ✳ Information   Gluten-free, wheat-free, nut-free. Contains soy.

GARNISHES

Garnishes in the lunch box? You bet!

Nothing makes a packed lunch seem more special than the "touch of fancy" a garnish brings. Taking one or two extra moments in the morning to tuck a little garnish into a packed lunch makes an everyday lunch feel like a treat.

In addition to the garnish recipes in this chapter, other simple garnish ideas include . . .

- A slice or wedge of lemon or lime (in addition to being pretty, lemon and lime can also help mask the smell of strong-smelling foods in the lunch box; this is especially handy when packing brassicas like broccoli, cauliflower, and brussels sprouts)
- Fresh herbs (parsley, dill, mint, basil, rosemary, etc.)
- Edible flowers
- Green pea tendrils
- Carrot, daikon, jicama, bell pepper, or cucumber slices cut into decorative shapes using a sharp knife or cookie cutters

- A strip of citrus peel or small strip of carrot, tied in a knot
- Melon balls on small food picks

Nonfood items can also act as lunchtime special touches:

- Decorative toothpicks or food picks
- Small squirt bottles filled with dressing or soy sauce
- A pretty napkin
- A handwritten note

BANDERILLAS

Quick & Easy

(Spain)

Nothing could be easier or faster than preparing this traditional *tapas* from Spain. Feel free to substitute other ingredients such as marinated mushrooms or pepperoncini.

3 or 4 make a good serving

Special equipment you will need:
Toothpicks or food picks

1 jar cocktail onions
1 jar small sweet gherkin pickles
1 jar pitted green olives, stuffed with pimento

▸ Alternate cocktail onions, gherkins, and green olives on the food picks or toothpicks, three or four items per pick.

Allergen Information ✳ Gluten-free, wheat-free, soy-free, nut-free.

CARROT AND DAIKON FLOWERS

These little garnishes don't have to be flowers; they can just as easily be hearts, stars, or other shapes. Use small cookie cutters or look for cutters designed especially for vegetables at gourmet food shops or online.

Makes several
flowers

Special equipment you will need:
Small cookie cutters (preferably sharp
    stainless steel) or vegetable cutters

1 wide carrot or daikon radish

▸ Peel the carrot or daikon and slice crosswise into paper-thin slices. Use a cutter to cut the slices into flowers or other decorative shapes.

Allergen ✳ Gluten-free, wheat-free,
Information   soy-free, nut-free.

CARROT-CUCUMBER TULIPS

Use these cuties to decorate your lunch boxes or veggie platters.

Makes several
tulips

1 medium cucumber
1 medium carrot
Toothpicks (preferably green)

▸ Slice the cucumber into ½-inch rounds. Slice the rounds in half. Use a sharp knife to remove the seeds and trim the inside edges to look like two petals.

- Peel the carrot and slice into ½-inch rounds. Use your knife to cut two V-shaped wedges out of one side of the carrot round, to resemble a tulip.
- Poke the toothpick through the middle of the cucumber petals and top with the carrot tulip.

Allergen ✳ Information   Gluten-free, wheat-free, soy-free, nut-free.

CHILE BLOSSOM

A pretty garnish for spicy dishes like curry. Make sure to use gloves and avoid touching your eyes when handling hot chiles.

Makes 1 blossom

1 small, narrow, long, red or green chile

- Using scissors, cut the chile lengthwise from the top, leaving at least 1 inch at the base of the chile uncut. Cut down the chile about six or eight times, forming six to eight "petals."
- Carefully scrape out the seeds and ribs. Place the chile in a bowl of ice water for at least one hour, or until the "petals" are curling out.

Allergen ✳ Information   Gluten-free, wheat-free, soy-free, nut-free.

OCTO-CELERY

A very common addition to Japanese bento boxes is the "octo-dog"—a hotdog cut and cooked to resemble an octopus. Unfortunately, vegan hotdogs don't "curl" when cooked, so they don't make very good octo-dogs. Happily, celery curls and makes a fine octopus, and a much healthier one, too.

Makes 1
octo-celery

1 stalk celery

Black sesame seeds for eyes and mouth
   (optional)

▸ Prepare a bowl of ice water and set aside.

▸ Trim the ends off the celery stalk and cut off a 3-inch section.

▸ Take the section and use a sharp knife to cut from one end lengthwise to just past center. Repeat, creating eight thin strips of celery (the octopus "legs").

▸ Place the celery in the bowl of ice water and refrigerate until the ends curl, several hours or overnight.

▸ Use a toothpick to poke holes in the celery for eyes and a mouth, and wedge black sesame seeds into the holes.

Allergen Information ✳ Gluten-free, wheat-free, soy-free, nut-free.

RADISH ROSETTES

Why eat plain old radishes when you could be eating radish rosettes? I felt so clever when I first discovered how to make these. For a while I kept a constant bowl of ice water filled with radish rosettes in my refrigerator and garnished my every plate with them.

Makes several radish rosettes

1 bunch large red radishes

▶ Cut off the bottom and top ends of a radish, so it stands up and has a clean round top.
▶ Set the radish upright on a cutting board and use a sharp paring knife to cut four thin vertical slices evenly spaced down the sides of the radish; these are the "petals." Cut straight down, stopping about three-quarters of the way down the side of the radish.
▶ The petals should be thin and slightly loose to the touch, or they will not "open," so make your petals as thin as you can without cutting all the way through.
▶ Immerse the radishes in a bowl of ice water and refrigerate for at least one hour, long enough for the "petals" to spread open slightly.

VARIATIONS:

▶ Double the petals by making another set behind the first set, about ⅛ inch in from the first.
▶ Make six smaller petals instead of four.
▶ Make angled petals by using two knife strokes to make each petal, angling the tip of your knife slightly inward at the center of each petal.
▶ Decorate the top of the radish by cutting V-shaped wedges all along the top, angling the cuts in toward the center.

Allergen Information ✳ Gluten-free, wheat-free, soy-free, nut-free.

CHAPTER

17

SALADS AND DRESSINGS

BASIL SALAD WITH LIME AND RED CURRY DRESSING

(Thailand)

This salad gets its spark from snappy Thai basil and red curry paste. Pack the dressing in a separate container and dress the salad just before serving.

Makes 2 servings

1 cucumber

1 head romaine lettuce, washed, dried, and
    chopped into bite-size pieces

1 tablespoon fresh Thai basil (or regular basil),
    cut into thin ribbons, plus extra for garnish

1 tablespoon cilantro, minced, plus extra for
    garnish

1 tablespoon freshly squeezed lime juice

1 teaspoon Thai red curry paste (I use
    Thai Kitchen Red Curry Paste)

2 teaspoons toasted sesame oil

1 teaspoon sugar

Pinch of salt, or to taste

▸ Peel the cucumber, then use the peeler to slice the cucumber into long ribbons, leaving off when you get to the soft seeded center. Discard the seeds.

▸ Toss the cucumber with the lettuce, Thai basil, and cilantro.

▸ To make the dressing, whisk the lime juice, red curry paste, sesame oil, sugar, and salt together in a small bowl. Add the dressing to the salad just before serving.

Allergen ✳ Information   Gluten-free, wheat-free, soy-free, nut-free.

BEAN SPROUT SALAD

(Korea)

Blanching the mung bean sprouts cooks them slightly but leaves them crunchy.

Makes 2 servings

1½ cups fresh mung bean sprouts

½ teaspoon low-sodium soy sauce

1 teaspoon rice vinegar

½ teaspoon toasted sesame oil

½ teaspoon sugar

Pinch of cayenne, or to taste

Salt and freshly ground black pepper,
    to taste

2 scallions, sliced (white and part of
    the green)

▸ Fill a large bowl with ice water and set aside.
▸ Blanch the bean sprouts: bring a large saucepan of water to a boil. Add the bean sprouts and cook for 2 minutes, until crisp-tender. Immediately plunge the bean sprouts into the ice water. Drain well and place in a bowl.
▸ In a small bowl combine the soy sauce, vinegar, sesame oil, sugar, cayenne, and salt and pepper. Stir until the sugar dissolves. Drizzle over the bean sprouts and toss. Top with sliced scallions.

Allergen ✳ Information   Gluten-free, wheat-free, nut-free. Contains soy.

BEET SALAD

(Germany)

I love pickled beets! These taste better than canned beets and have the added flavor of caraway seeds.

Makes 4 servings

1 bunch beets, washed and trimmed but
   not peeled
2 tablespoons white wine vinegar
1 tablespoon olive oil
½ teaspoon sugar
Pinch of ground cloves
Salt and freshly ground black pepper, to taste
½ teaspoon caraway seeds (optional)

▸ Place the whole, unpeeled beets in a medium saucepan and fill with water to cover. Bring to a boil, then lower the heat and simmer, partially covered, until beets are tender, about 45 minutes to 1 hour, depending on the size.

▸ Drain the beets. When the beets are cool enough to handle, remove the skin with the back of a paring knife and dice or slice. Place the sliced beets in a small mixing bowl.

▸ In another small bowl whisk together 2 tablespoons water with the vinegar, olive oil, sugar, cloves, and salt and pepper.

▸ If you like the taste of caraway, grind the seeds briefly in a spice grinder or with a mortar and pestle and add to the dressing.

▸ Pour the dressing over the beets and marinate, refrigerated, for several hours before serving.

Allergen Information ✳ Gluten-free, wheat-free, soy-free, nut-free.

BROCCOLI SALAD WITH DAIKON FLOWERS

(Japan)

Crisp-tender broccoli is topped with a sesame-soy sauce dressing and decorated with delicate daikon radish flowers.

Makes 4 servings

5 cups broccoli, cut into small florets

2 tablespoons tahini (sesame paste)

3 tablespoons low-sodium soy sauce

1 tablespoon sugar

Toasted sesame seeds

Daikon Flowers (page 69) for garnish

▸ Have a bowl of ice water ready. Bring a medium saucepan filled with water to a boil. Add the broccoli florets and simmer until crisp-tender, about 3 minutes. Immediately drain the broccoli and plunge into the ice water, then drain again.

▸ Mix together the tahini, soy sauce, and sugar and pour some over the broccoli. Divide the broccoli into four bowls or lunch containers. Sprinkle each serving with toasted sesame seeds and arrange Daikon Flowers over the top.

Allergen ✳ Information Gluten-free, wheat-free, nut-free. Contains soy.

CARIBBEAN COLESLAW

This is a super-quick coleslaw with the sweetness of pineapple and the tang of fresh lime. It tastes best after sitting for at least an hour to allow the flavors to marry.

Makes 4 servings

8 ounces packaged shredded coleslaw mix
   (about 4 cups mixed shredded green
   and red cabbage and carrots)
1 (8-ounce) can pineapple tidbits, with
   their juice
1 teaspoon fresh lime zest
2 tablespoons freshly squeezed lime juice
Salt, to taste

▸ Combine the cabbage mix, pineapple, lime zest, and lime juice and toss to combine. Season with salt. Chill at least 1 hour before serving.

Allergen ✳ Information   Gluten-free, wheat-free, soy-free, nut-free.

CARROT AND DAIKON SALAD

(Japan)

This salad is one of my favorite ways to enjoy daikon. Daikon are giant white radishes that look like large carrots; they have a mild, sweet flavor and are not as spicy as small red radishes.

Makes 4 servings

2 medium carrots

1 medium daikon

Salt, to taste

2 tablespoons brown rice vinegar

¾ teaspoon sugar

1½ teaspoons low-sodium soy sauce

▸ Peel the carrot and daikon and cut them into matchsticks. Spread them out together in a thin layer on a large platter and sprinkle lightly with salt. Refrigerate for 30 minutes, then pat them dry with a kitchen towel and place in a medium bowl.

▸ Mix together the vinegar, sugar, and soy sauce. Pour over the carrots and daikon and toss to coat.

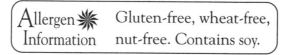 Allergen Information — Gluten-free, wheat-free, nut-free. Contains soy.

CUCUMBER TOMATO SALAD

If you're making this for a Greek meal, add some Kalamata olives, a few slices of red onion, and a sprinkle of dried oregano. Splurge on a good-quality extra virgin olive oil for this salad; it makes a difference.

Makes 4 servings

4 large fresh tomatoes, seeded and cut into
   bite-size pieces
1 large cucumber, peeled and cut into
   bite-size pieces
½ cup fresh parsley, minced
3 tablespoons olive oil
1½ tablespoons freshly squeezed lemon juice
Salt and freshly ground black pepper, to taste

▸ Toss the tomatoes, cucumbers, and parsley together in a serving bowl.

▸ In a small bowl, whisk together the olive oil, lemon juice, and salt and pepper. Drizzle over the salad just before serving.

Allergen Information ✳ Gluten-free, wheat-free, soy-free, nut-free.

CURTIDO

(El Salvador)

This spicy slaw is traditionally served with Pupusas (page 129).

(page 129)

Makes 4 to 6 servings

½ head green cabbage, chopped into coarse shreds (about 6 cups)

1 large carrot, peeled and grated

1 jalapeño, seeded and minced

3 scallions, sliced

¼ cup white distilled vinegar

1 tablespoon olive oil

½ teaspoon dried oregano

1 teaspoon sugar

⅛ teaspoon cayenne (optional, or to taste)

Salt, to taste

▸ Bring a large saucepan filled with water to a boil. Place the cabbage and carrot in a heat-proof mixing bowl and pour in the boiling water, covering the cabbage. Let stand for 2 minutes. Drain in a colander. When cool enough to handle, press out as much liquid as possible.

▸ Place the cabbage back in the mixing bowl and add the jalapeño and scallions. Whisk together the vinegar, olive oil, oregano, sugar, cayenne (if using), and salt. Pour the dressing over the cabbage and toss to combine. Chill.

Allergen ✳ Information — Gluten-free, wheat-free, soy-free, nut-free.

PICNIC POTATO SALAD

I love this mayo-free version of potato salad. This makes a great potluck or picnic dish.

Makes 8 servings

3 pounds Yukon Gold potatoes (about 8)

¼ cup apple cider vinegar

¼ cup olive oil

1 medium red onion, diced

2 tablespoons Dijon mustard

3 tablespoons capers

1 bell pepper (any color), seeded and diced

4 stalks of celery, chopped

Salt and freshly ground black pepper,
    to taste

▸ Boil the potatoes in their skins until tender but still holding their shape, about 20 to 25 minutes. Drain. As soon as the potatoes are cool enough to handle, peel the skins off with the back of a knife. Dice the potatoes, place them in a mixing bowl, and add the vinegar.

▸ Heat the olive oil in a sauté pan and cook the onion, stirring often, until barely soft, about 3 minutes. Add to the potatoes along with the mustard, capers, bell pepper, and celery. Season with salt and pepper.

Allergen ✳ Information   Gluten-free, wheat-free, soy-free, nut-free.

STICKS-AND-STONES SALAD

Kid Friendly

I think the name alone might entice kids to give this salad a try! Blanching the celery and carrot sticks changes their texture just a touch, leaving them crunchy but tastier than raw. The dressing is fantastic; don't forget the dill.

Makes 4 servings

----
2 cups celery sticks (about 1½ inches in length)

1 cup carrot sticks (about 1½ inches in length)

1 (8-ounce) can whole water chestnuts, drained and rinsed

2 tablespoons olive oil

2 tablespoons apple cider vinegar

1 teaspoon Dijon-style mustard

¼ teaspoon dried dill weed

½ teaspoon sugar

Salt, to taste

▸ Blanch the celery and carrot sticks: bring a medium saucepan filled with water to a boil. Add the celery and carrot sticks and cook, uncovered, for 3 minutes. Drain and immediately rinse the sticks with cold water.

▸ Place the celery and carrot sticks in a bowl with the water chestnuts.

▸ In a small bowl, whisk together the olive oil, vinegar, mustard, dill, sugar, and salt. Pour over the "sticks and stones" and toss to coat.

Allergen Information ✳ Gluten-free, wheat-free, soy-free, nut-free.

THAI CUCUMBER SALAD

(Thailand)

This simple cucumber salad is served often in Thai cuisine. It re-freshes and soothes the palate when the rest of the meal is spicy.

For lunch planning, make the dressing the night before and refrigerate, then pour over the cucumbers just before packing.

Makes 4 servings

¼ cup rice vinegar

1½ tablespoons sugar

2 medium cucumbers

½ small red onion, peeled and very
thinly sliced

Salt, to taste

▸ Combine the vinegar and sugar in a small saucepan and bring to a boil, stirring with a wooden spoon until the sugar is no longer visible. Reduce heat and simmer for 2 to 3 minutes, or until sugar has dissolved completely and the vinegar has reduced slightly.

▸ Transfer the vinegar dressing to a small bowl and refrigerate until completely cool.

▸ Peel the cucumbers and use a mandoline or sharp knife to slice into very thin rounds. Toss with the red onion and dressing. Season with salt.

Allergen ✳ Information   Gluten-free, wheat-free, soy-free, nut-free.

SANDWICHES AND WRAPS

BAGUETTE WITH ROASTED RED PEPPER SPREAD

Quick & Easy

You can have these sandwiches ready for a picnic or lunch in a snap. The creamy roasted pepper spread pairs nicely with the softness of the baguette and the crisp crunch of fresh vegetables.

Makes 4 sandwiches	1 18-inch French-bread baguette

1 recipe Roasted Red Pepper Spread
  (page 65)

½ to ¾ cup cucumber, peeled, seeded,
  and diced

8 romaine lettuce leaves

2 cups thinly sliced radicchio

- Cut the loaf of baguette bread crosswise into four equal pieces. Cut each piece horizontally in half. Scoop out some of the center from each piece of bread, making space for the fillings.
- Spread the Roasted Red Pepper Spread on the bottom halves of bread. Top with cucumber, lettuce, and radicchio and cover with the other slice of bread.

Allergen ✳ Information — Nut-free. Contains gluten, wheat, and soy.

CAPONATA SANDWICHES

(Italy)

Caponata is a famous dish from Sicily. There are many, many variations; this one has an added touch of sweetness from raisins. If you like vegan mozzarella, add a slice or two to your sandwich; if not, the sandwich is just as good without.

Makes 4 to 6 sandwiches

2 tablespoons olive oil

1 medium onion, diced

1 stalk celery, chopped

1 medium eggplant, cut into 1-inch cubes

1 red, yellow, or orange bell pepper, seeded and chopped

1 (14.5-ounce) can diced tomatoes, drained

1 teaspoon dried basil

½ teaspoon dried oregano

¼ cup raisins

2 tablespoons red wine vinegar

2 tablespoons sugar

Salt and freshly ground black pepper,
    to taste

1 loaf ciabatta bread (or other crusty,
    artisan-style bread)

Vegan mozzarella slices (optional)

▸ Heat the olive oil in a large saucepan over medium-high heat. Add the onion, celery, eggplant, and bell pepper, and cook, stirring frequently, until the eggplant starts to soften, about 5 minutes.

▸ Add the drained canned tomatoes, basil, oregano, and raisins. Turn the heat to low, cover, and simmer for 25 minutes, stirring occasionally, until eggplant is tender.

▸ Add the vinegar and sugar along with salt and pepper. Let cool.

▸ Cut the loaf of ciabatta bread into 3- to 4-inch wedges and cut the wedges in half. Toast the bread in a dry skillet and fill with caponata (or you may want to pack the caponata separately and fill the sandwiches at lunchtime).

▸ Top the caponata with slices of vegan mozzarella if desired.

Allergen ✳ Information   The caponata mixture itself is gluten-free, wheat-free, soy-free, and nut-free. The sandwiches contain gluten and wheat (in the bread) and soy (in the vegan mozzarella.)

MY FAVORITE TOFURKY SANDWICH

This is my favorite thing to do with leftover Tofurky and cranberry sauce after Thanksgiving. If it's not that time of year, this recipe will also taste just as good with regular Tofurky deli slices.

Makes 1 sandwich

Vegenaise

2 slices sourdough sandwich bread
   (or white or wheat)

Salt and freshly ground black pepper,
   to taste

2 teaspoons cranberry sauce, or more
   to taste

2 or 3 slices of leftover Tofurky Roast
   with stuffing

▸ Spread Vegenaise on both slices of bread and top with salt and pepper as desired. Spread a layer of cranberry sauce on top of the Vegenaise on one slice of the bread.

▸ Top the bread with slices of Tofurky and stuffing. Cover with the other bread slice, cut in half, and pack or serve.

Allergen Information ✳ Nut-free. Contains gluten, wheat, and soy.

PLANTAIN WRAPS WITH TANGY BLACK BEAN SPREAD

For this recipe, look for ripe plantains with skins that are dark yellow with black patches.

Makes 4 servings

2 ripe plantains

2 tablespoons canola oil

Salt and freshly ground black pepper, to taste

4 10-inch round wraps or tortillas

1 recipe Tangy Black Bean Spread (page 66)

Salsa for serving

▸ Use a sharp knife to cut the stems off the plantains and peel the skin off. Cut the plantains in half, then cut each half into quarters lengthwise.

▸ Heat the oil in a large nonstick or well-seasoned cast-iron skillet over medium heat. When hot add the plantains in a single layer. Fry the plantains on one side until the side turns a reddish brown, about 5 minutes. Turn and repeat on all sides.

▸ Transfer the fried plantains to a paper towel to drain. Sprinkle with salt and pepper.

▸ Heat the wraps or tortillas briefly on both sides in a warm dry skillet to soften them and make them pliable. Spread each wrap with Black Bean Spread, fill with four fried plantain wedges, and roll up like a burrito, tucking the ends in as you go.

▸ Serve with salsa for dipping.

Allergen ✳ Information Nut-free. Contains gluten and wheat (in the wrap) and soy (in the bean spread).

VEGEMITE SANDWICH

(Australia)

Americans, don't freak out on me! Vegemite is a dark, savory yeast extract that has a salty, "beefy" taste that reminds me of strong miso. It's really quite good!

Makes 1 sandwich

2 slices sandwich bread, white or wheat

Nonhydrogenated margarine

Vegemite

Lettuce leaves

Freshly sliced tomato

Freshly sliced cucumber

Freshly sliced avocado (optional)

▸ Toast the bread. Spread each piece of bread with a thin layer of margarine. Spread a thin layer of Vegemite over the margarine on one piece of the bread.

▸ Layer lettuce, tomato, cucumber, avocado, and more lettuce on the slice of bread. Top with the other piece of bread, cut in half, and pack or serve.

Allergen Information ❋ Soy-free, nut-free. Contains gluten and wheat.

VIETNAMESE SALAD ROLLS

Rice paper wrappers make wonderful gluten-free sandwich wrappers. In this recipe the rice paper is wrapped around meaty, seared portobello mushrooms, rice noodles, and fresh, flavorful herbs.

To make preparation fast and easy in the morning, prepare the Asian Portobellos, lettuce, and herbs the night before and refrigerate. In the morning, prepare the noodles and wrap the rolls.

Look for rice vermicelli noodles, rice paper wrappers, and hoisin sauce in the Asian section at your grocery store or at an Asian market.

Makes 8 rolls	2 ounces rice vermicelli noodles

Makes 8 rolls

2 ounces rice vermicelli noodles

8 rice wrappers (8.5-inch diameter)

1 recipe Asian Portobellos (page 161), cooled completely

2 tablespoons roughly chopped fresh Thai basil (or regular basil)

1 tablespoon roughly chopped fresh mint leaves

3 tablespoons roughly chopped fresh cilantro

2 cups leaf or butterhead lettuce leaves, chopped, plus 8 whole lettuce leaves for serving

Hoisin sauce for serving

Dry roasted peanuts, finely chopped (optional)

▸ To prepare the noodles, bring a medium saucepan of water to boil. Add the noodles and cook until they are white and al dente, about 3 to 5 minutes. Drain the noodles, rinse well in cold water, and drain again. Set the noodles aside.

- Fill a large bowl with warm water. Dip one wrapper into the hot water for 5 seconds, or until softened. Transfer the rice wrapper to a dry work surface and pat dry.
- Arrange a handful of vermicelli, slices of portobello, basil, mint, cilantro, and chopped lettuce in a mound just below the center of the wrapper. Roll up the rice paper to form a tight bundle, folding in the sides along the way.
- Serve or pack each salad roll wrapped in a lettuce leaf (this will keep them from sticking to the plate or packing container). If packing for later, cover the rolls with plastic wrap to keep them from drying out.
- Serve with hoisin sauce for dipping, mixing some chopped peanuts into the hoisin if you like.
- These rolls should be eaten the same day they are made. Don't re-frigerate them; the rice paper may dry out.

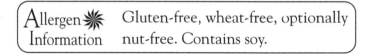

Allergen Information — Gluten-free, wheat-free, optionally nut-free. Contains soy.

SOUPS AND STEWS

HOT NOODLE SOUP

Chicken Noodle's got nothing on this soup! It's so warm and comforting, the perfect soup for a day when you're feeling under the weather. It cooks in mere minutes, another plus if you're not feeling well.

Makes 2 to 3 servings

2 medium tomatoes, peeled and diced fine (page xiv)

1 clove garlic, minced

1 vegan chicken-flavored bouillon cube

2 teaspoons fresh ginger, grated

¼ cup fresh cilantro, roughly chopped

1 jalapeño, cut in half and seeded (optional, this makes it spicy but really clears out the sinuses)

½ teaspoon ground cumin

½ teaspoon freshly ground black pepper

2 ounces dried angel hair pasta noodles, broken into 2-inch pieces

2 teaspoons canola oil

¼ teaspoon whole black mustard seeds

- In a medium saucepan, combine 4 cups water, the tomatoes, garlic, bouillon cube, ginger, cilantro, jalapeño (if using), cumin, and pepper. Bring to a boil, turn the heat to low and simmer for 8 minutes. Add the angel hair noodles during the last 4 minutes of cooking.
- Heat the canola oil in a small skillet over medium-high heat. Add the mustard seeds, cover and cook until the seeds sizzle and pop, about 30 seconds. Scrape the oil and seeds into the soup. Remove the jalapeño before serving.

> Allergen ✳ Information   Soy-free, nut-free. Contains gluten and wheat.

MARTIE'S GUMBO

(New Orleans)

Martie, a fine vegan from Louisiana, was kind enough to invite our local vegetarian group into her home one day to show us how to make (and eat!) her delicious vegan version of traditional Cajun Gumbo. Martie says to leave out the vegan sausage, if you prefer, for an Okra and Tomato Gumbo that is just as tasty. Serve this stew over rice (two parts gumbo to one part rice is about right).

Makes 6 servings

¼ cup all-purpose flour

¼ cup plus 1 tablespoon canola oil

1 large onion, chopped

½ green bell pepper, chopped

1 stalk celery, chopped

1 tablespoon minced garlic

1 (16-ounce) package frozen chopped okra

1 (28-ounce) can diced tomatoes

Salt, to taste

1 (14-ounce) package Tofurky Italian
    Sausage or one 14-ounce package
    Lightlife Gimme Lean Sausage (optional),
    cut into bite-size pieces

½ cup fresh parsley, minced

1 bunch scallions, whites and part of the
    green, chopped

Optional seasonings, to taste: cayenne,
    Tabasco sauce, Cajun seasoning
    blend, and/or Gumbo Filé (dried
    sassafras leaves)

- First, make the Cajun Roux: mix the flour and ¼ cup oil together in a large saucepan over medium low heat. Stir the mixture constantly until the roux is a medium brown (about the color of a paper bag).
- Add the onion, green pepper, and celery and cook, stirring frequently, until the onion is soft. Add the garlic and cook, stirring, for another minute. Add the okra, the tomatoes with their liquid, salt, and 1½ quarts of water (you may need to add additional water while cooking to reach the desired consistency of a slightly thick soup).
- Bring to a boil over high heat, then reduce the heat to low and simmer, covered, for at least 1 hour (a Gumbo may cook all day in Louisiana, says Martie, and will taste increasingly better as it cooks).
- Meanwhile, brown the vegan sausage, if using, in a skillet with the remaining tablespoon canola oil. Add the vegan sausage to the gumbo during the last 45 minutes of cooking. Add the parsley and green onions during the last 30 minutes.
- Serve the gumbo over rice, and add any of the optional seasonings listed above, as desired.

Allergen ✳ Information   Nut-free, optionally soy-free. Contains gluten and wheat.

MOROCCAN TAGINE

(Morocco)

Serve this fragrant spiced stew over couscous, whole wheat couscous, or Orange Couscous (page 150) for a traditional Moroccan experience, or over quinoa for a gluten-free meal.

Wear kitchen gloves when peeling butternut squash: the skin exudes a sticky liquid as it is peeled.

Makes 6 servings

¼ teaspoon cinnamon

1 teaspoon ginger

1 teaspoon cumin

1 teaspoon paprika

¼ teaspoon turmeric

⅛ teaspoon cayenne

2 tablespoons olive oil

1 medium onion, peeled, halved, and cut
     into half-rings

½ medium yellow, orange, or red bell pepper,
     seeded and diced

1 (15-ounce) can diced tomatoes

1 medium butternut squash, peeled,
     seeded, and cut into 1-inch cubes
     (about 6 to 7 cups)

1 (15-ounce) can chickpeas, rinsed and
     drained

2 medium zucchini, cut in half lengthwise,
     then cut into ½-inch slices

½ cup golden or regular raisins

Salt, to taste

Chopped fresh parsley for garnish

- ▸ Measure out all the spices into one small dish and set aside.
- ▸ Heat the olive oil in a large saucepan over medium heat. Add the onions and cook, stirring occasionally, until the they are soft and translucent, about 7 minutes (adjust the heat as needed to keep them from browning). Add the bell pepper and all the spices and cook, stirring, for another minute.
- ▸ Add the diced tomatoes with all their juices, the butternut squash, and 2 cups of water. Bring to a boil, then reduce the heat to low and simmer, covered, for 20 minutes or until squash is almost tender.
- ▸ Add the chickpeas, zucchini, and raisins and continue to simmer, covered, for another 10 minutes, or until squash is tender. Season with salt. Garnish each serving with parsley just before serving.

Allergen ✳ Information   Gluten-free, wheat-free, soy-free, nut-free.

NEW ENGLAND CHOWDER

Using fresh corn to make corn "cream" gives this dish extra tenderness and flavor. To remove the kernels from a fresh ear of corn, set the corn cob on its end in a large mixing bowl and use a serrated bread knife to saw away the kernels. Then go around the cob with the other side of the knife (the dull back side of the blade), scraping down the sides of the corn cob to squeeze out the rest of the corn and its creamy "milk."

This comforting soup is the perfect thing tucked into an insulated food jar on a cold winter's day.

Makes 4 servings

2 cups fresh or thawed frozen corn kernels

3 tablespoons canola oil or nonhydrogenated
   margarine

1 large onion, peeled and diced

3 stalks celery, diced

2 medium carrots, peeled and diced

2 medium russet potatoes, peeled and cut
   in a ½-inch dice

½ teaspoon dried thyme

1 bay leaf

1 (3-ounce) can shiitake mushrooms or
   one 4-ounce can white mushroom pieces
   and stems, rinsed and drained

Salt and white pepper, to taste

▶ Place the corn kernels in a medium saucepan with 2 cups water. Bring to a boil and simmer for 15 minutes, until tender. Let the corn cool slightly, then pour the cooked corn and all the cooking liquid in a blender container and blend on high until smooth.

Strain the corn "milk" through a sieve to remove and discard any unblended fibers. Set the milk aside.

▸ Heat the oil or margarine in a large saucepan over medium high heat. Add the onion, celery, and carrots and cook, stirring frequently, until the onion is soft and translucent, about 7 minutes.

▸ Add 3 cups of water along with the diced potato, thyme, and bay leaf. Bring to a boil, turn heat to low, and simmer, covered, until potato is almost tender, about 8 to 9 minutes.

▸ Add the corn "cream," mushrooms, salt, and white pepper. Simmer for 1 to 2 more minutes, until potatoes are tender but not falling apart (mash a few of the potatoes against the side of the pan with a wooden spoon to thicken the chowder, if you like).

▸ Taste for seasonings and remove the bay leaf before serving.

Allergen ✳ Information   Gluten-free, wheat-free, soy-free, nut-free. Contains corn.

RATATOUILLE

(France)

Ratatouille tastes even better the day after it is made, making it perfect for lunch packed in an insulated food jar alongside a wedge of crusty baguette and a bit of dark chocolate.

I like to add canellini or other beans to my ratatouille for some extra protein, but the traditional dish does not contain them.

Makes 4 servings

2 tablespoons olive oil

1 medium onion, peeled and diced

3 cloves garlic, peeled and minced

½ yellow, red, or orange bell pepper, seeded and diced

1 large, firm purple eggplant, diced

3 large tomatoes, peeled and diced (see page xiv)

½ teaspoon dried thyme

1 teaspoon basil

3 medium zucchini, cut in half lengthwise, then cut into ½-inch slices

1 (15-ounce) can canellini or other beans, rinsed and drained (optional)

Salt and pepper, to taste

¼ cup fresh flat leaf parsley, minced

▸ Heat the olive oil in a large saucepan over medium heat. Add the onions and cook, stirring occasionally, until they are soft and translucent, about 7 minutes. Add the garlic and bell pepper and cook, stirring, for another minute (turn the heat down if the garlic is turning brown).

- Add the eggplant, tomatoes, thyme, and basil. Bring to a simmer. Turn the heat down and simmer, covered, for 15 minutes.
- Add the zucchini and beans and simmer, covered, for another 10 to 15 minutes, just until the zucchini is tender.
- Season with salt and pepper to your liking, and sprinkle with parsley just before serving.

Allergen Information ✳ Gluten-free, wheat-free, soy-free, nut-free.

VEGETARIAN PHO

(Vietnam)

You'll want to pack this pho in three separate containers: one pre-heated insulated food jar filled with the hot beef-flavored broth, a separate container filled with rice noodles, and another filled with your choice of garnishes.

When my son ate this pho during the testing for this cookbook he told me, "This is one of the best things I've ever tasted so far!"

Makes 4 servings

3 vegetarian beef-flavored bouillon cubes
   (I use Celifibr brand)

1¼-inch slice of fresh ginger

2 whole star anise

2 whole cloves

1 cardamom pod

1 2-inch cinnamon stick

8 ounces (about ½ tub) Chinese-style
   firm tofu, cut into ½-inch cubes

⅛ teaspoon freshly ground black pepper

1 cup fresh mung bean sprouts, rinsed and drained

3 ounces flat rice stick noodles (medium-size
   rice noodles that look like linguini, the same
   used for Pad Thai)

6 fresh scallions, sliced (white and part of
   the green)

1 fresh red or green chile, seeded and sliced
   into thin rounds

1 cup fresh cilantro, roughly chopped

1 cup fresh Thai basil leaves (or regular basil),
   roughly chopped

4 lime wedges

- To make the broth, bring 6 cups water, the bouillon cubes, ginger, anise, cloves, cardamom pod, and cinnamon stick to a boil in a large saucepan. Reduce heat and simmer for 15 minutes. Strain the broth into a clean saucepan and return to a boil. Add the tofu, pepper, and bean sprouts and cook for one more minute. Remove from heat.
- Meanwhile, to cook the rice noodles, bring a large pot of water to a boil. Remove from heat and add the noodles to the hot water. Soak the noodles, stirring occasionally with a fork to keep them from sticking together, until they are soft but al dente, about 7 minutes (or according to package directions). Drain the noodles immediately and rinse under cold water. Set aside.
- To serve, divide the noodles into four bowls. Ladle hot broth over the noodles and let the eaters sprinkle their bowls with scallions, fresh chile, cilantro, basil, and squeezes of fresh lime juice, as desired.

Allergen Information ✳ Gluten-free, wheat-free, nut-free. Contains soy.

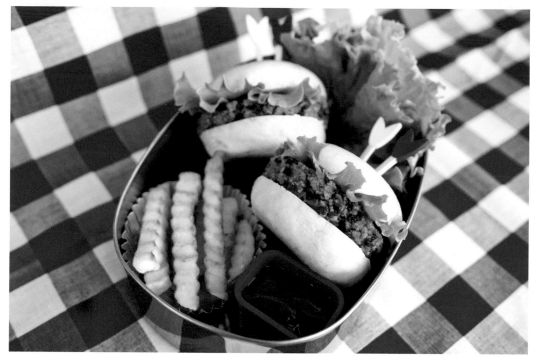

Kansas: Mini Veggie Burgers (page 126) on Mini Burger Buns (page 196) with french fries and ketchup.

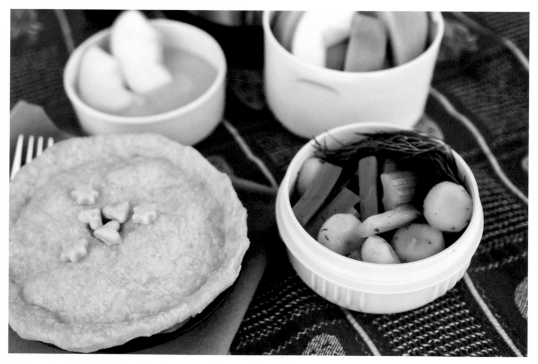

Nebraska: Chik'n Pot Pie (page 113), Sticks-and-Stones Salad (page 83), and apples with Caramel Dip (page 59).

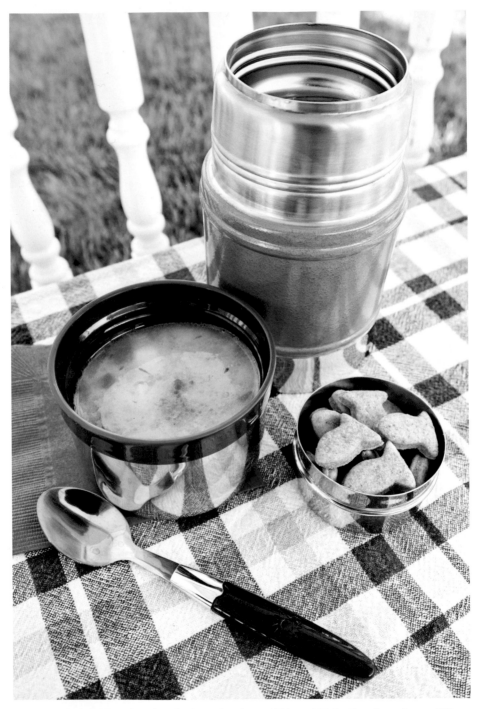

New England: New England Chowder (page 99) and Fish Crackers (page 53).

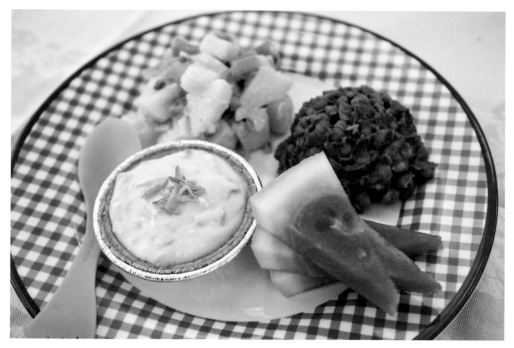

Picnic Time: Picnic Potato Salad (page 82), Barbecue Baked Beans (page 142), watermelon, and Coconut Cream Pielettes (page 219).

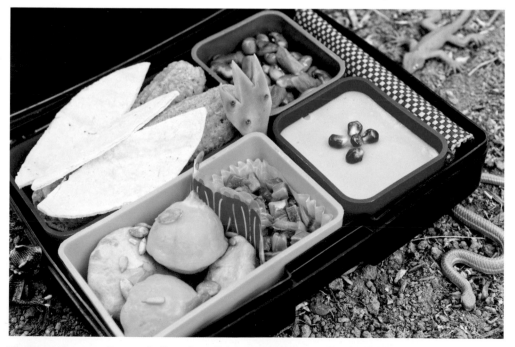

The Southwest: Corncob Cornbread (page 189) in tortilla "husks," Anasazi Beans (page 139), Prickly Pear Pudding (page 229), Fried Nopales (page 167), and Baby Squash Medley (page 162).

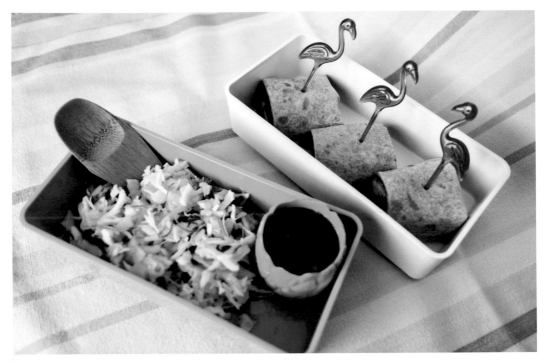

Caribbean #1: Plantain Wrap with Tangy Black Bean Spread (page 89), salsa, and Caribbean Coleslaw (page 78).

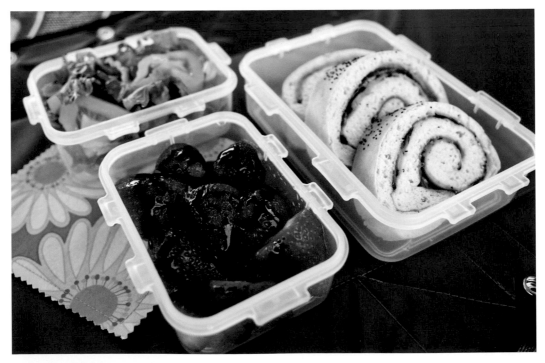

Italy #1: Grilled Vegetable Stromboli (page 193), Balsamic Strawberries (page 206), and green salad.

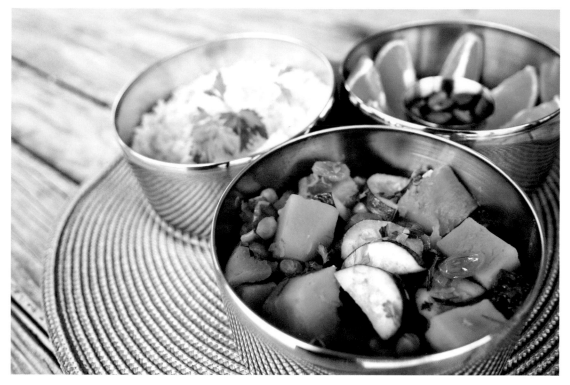

Morocco: Moroccan Tagine (page 97), Orange Couscous (page 150), tangerines, and Cinnamon-Sugar Almonds (page 51).

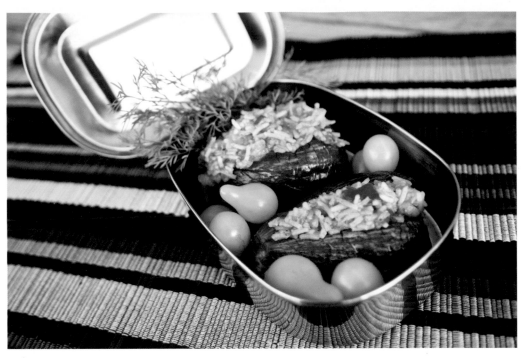

Turkey: Stuffed Eggplants (page 131) surrounded by yellow pear tomatoes.

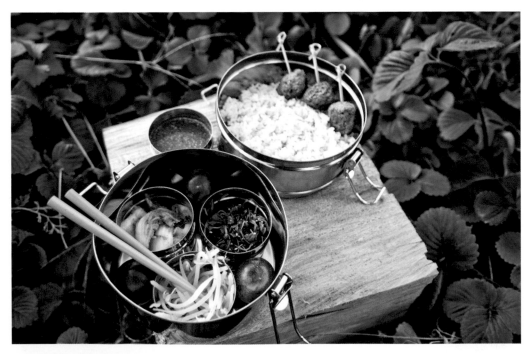

Korea: (clockwise from bottom) Bean Sprout Salad (page 75), plums, kimchi, Stir-Fried Watercress (page 181), Korean Dipping Sauce (page 61), Rice with Toasted Millet (page 153), and vegan meatballs.

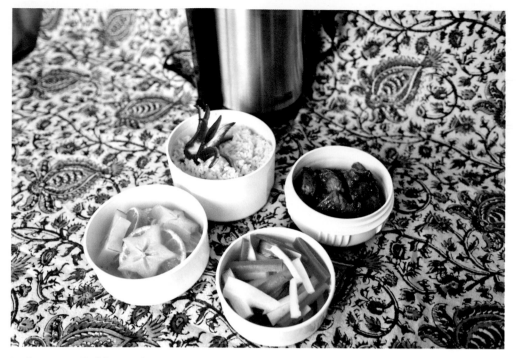

Indonesia: Golden Indonesian Tempeh (page 117), Indonesian Vegetable Pickles (page 169), tangerine and star fruit, and Yellow Coconut Rice (page 156).

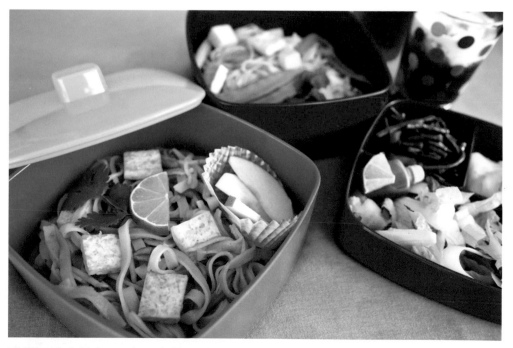

Thailand: (clockwise from left) Pad Thai (page 38), sliced Asian Pear, Mango Noodles (page 124), Thai Iced Tea (page 242), Red Curry Vegetables (page 176), Thai Cucumber Salad (page 84), and Basil Salad with Lime and Red Curry Dressing (page 73).

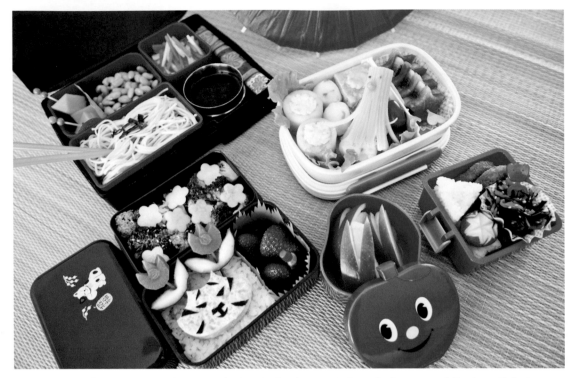

Japan: (in red Laptop Lunch System) Zaru Soba (page 136) with Carrot and Daikon Salad (page 79), edamame, and persimmon; (in pink bento) Tofu Tamagoyaki (page 133) with Potato Salad Balls (page 58), Octo-Celery (page 71), Cucumber Sushi Rolls (page 52), cherry tomatoes, kiwi and watermelon stars, and a Botan Rice Candy; (in red Gel-Cool bento box) Onigiri (page 148), vegan chicken nuggets, Stir-Fried Arame with Carrots and Ginger (page 179), Radish Rosettes (page 72), and (in red apple container) Apple Bunnies (page 203); (in kitty bento) Tofu Tiger (page 134), Carrot-Cucumber Tulips (page 69), Broccoli Salad with Daikon Flowers (page 77), and strawberries.

See Recommended Resources, page 247, for lunch box sources.

MAINS

BAHAMA MAMA'S BEANS AND RICE

Cooking beans and rice with coconut milk and spices is a common practice in the Caribbean. It transforms a simple dish into a filling meal that is rich, satisfying, and flavorful. Be careful when handling the Scotch Bonnet or any hot pepper—wear disposable gloves, wash your hands, and avoid touching your face.

Makes 4 servings

----

1 tablespoon canola oil

2 cloves garlic, minced

½ Scotch Bonnet or other hot pepper, seeded (optional)

1 (15-ounce) can black beans, rinsed and drained

1 cup dry long-grain white rice

½ cup coconut milk

4 scallions, chopped (white and part of the green)

½ teaspoon ground thyme

⅛ teaspoon cinnamon

⅛ teaspoon allspice

Salt and freshly ground black pepper,
     to taste

▶ Heat the oil in a medium saucepan over medium-high heat. Add the garlic and the optional pepper and cook, stirring, until the garlic is soft, about 1 minute.

▶ Add 1½ cups water to the saucepan along with the beans, rice, coconut milk, scallions, thyme, cinnamon, allspice, salt, and pepper. Bring to a boil, then turn the heat to low, cover, and simmer for 20 minutes. Take the saucepan off the heat and let the rice sit, still covered, for another 15 minutes.

▶ Taste for salt and remove the Scotch Bonnet pepper before serving.

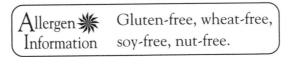

Allergen Information ✳ Gluten-free, wheat-free, soy-free, nut-free.

BLACK-EYED PEAS AND POTATOES WITH CILANTRO AND LIME

(Africa)

Protein-rich black-eyed peas are seasoned with cilantro, cumin, and lime in this hearty dish from Tanzania.

Makes 4 to 6 servings

2 tablespoons canola oil

3 cloves garlic, minced

1 teaspoon chili powder

1 tablespoon ground cumin

1 tablespoon ground coriander

1 teaspoon turmeric

1 (16-ounce) package frozen
    black-eyed peas

3 medium red potatoes, scrubbed
    and cut into bite-size pieces
    (about 3 cups)

2 tablespoons freshly squeezed
    lime juice

3 tablespoons fresh cilantro, minced

Salt, to taste

▸ Heat the canola oil in a large saucepan over medium heat. Add the garlic and cook, stirring, until the garlic is soft and fragrant, about 1 minute (adjust the heat down as needed if the garlic is cooking too fast and starting to brown).

▸ Add the chili powder, cumin, coriander, and turmeric and cook, stirring, for 1 more minute.

▸ Add the black-eyed peas and potatoes along with 1 cup water. Bring to a boil, lower the heat, and simmer, covered, until the potatoes are tender, about 10 to 12 minutes (add a bit more water if the liquid has cooked down and the potatoes are not tender yet; you want the dish to be thicker than a regular soup or stew).

▸ Stir in the lime juice, cilantro, and salt.

Allergen ✳ Information — Gluten-free, wheat-free, soy-free, nut-free.

CABBAGE ROLLS

These tasty little cabbage parcels are filled with a vegan loaf mixture made from nuts, beans, and rice. It makes a fantastic vegan centerpiece dish during the holidays.

This dish can be made in advance and refrigerated; it reheats well.

Makes 10 cabbage rolls

----

1 cup walnuts

1 cup canned chickpeas, rinsed and drained

1 cup cooked brown rice

1 cup oat bran

½ teaspoon marjoram

¼ teaspoon thyme

¼ teaspoon onion powder

2 tablespoons soy sauce

2 tablespoons Dijon-style mustard

18 to 20 large cabbage leaves

1 cup low sodium tomato-vegetable
    juice blend

2 tablespoons freshly squeezed lemon juice

Salt and freshly ground black pepper,
    to taste

- Preheat the oven to 350°F.
- Using a food processor fitted with the metal blade, process the walnuts into very small bits. Pour out the walnuts into a large mixing bowl and set aside.
- Add the chickpeas and brown rice to the bowl of the food processor and process until the mixture forms a coarse mash. Add to the mixing bowl along with the oat bran, marjoram, thyme, onion powder, soy sauce, and mustard. Using your hands, knead the mixture well until it is thoroughly mixed and holds its shape. Set aside.
- Bring a large saucepan of salted water to a boil. Add the cabbage leaves and cook for 2 to 3 minutes (the leaves should be limp enough to roll but not cooked through). Drain the leaves thoroughly.
- Place a cabbage leaf on your work surface (if there is a rip in the leaf, cover it with another small cabbage leaf; if the leaf has a tough middle stem that won't roll, cut it away and overlap the remaining leaf).
- Divide the bean and rice mixture into ten equal pieces. Scoop up one piece and form it into a tiny round loaf. Place the mixture at one edge of the cabbage leaf and roll it up, folding in the edges as you go.
- Place the cabbage rolls, seam side down, side-by-side in an oiled baking dish. Use a knife to shred all the remaining cabbage leaves and pieces you have left over. Sprinkle it over and around the cabbage rolls.
- Mix the tomato juice and lemon juice together and pour evenly over the rolls. Sprinkle with salt and pepper. Bake the rolls for 45 to 50 minutes, until gently brown on top.

Allergen ❋ Information   Gluten-free, wheat-free. Contains soy and nuts.

CALIFORNIA ROLL

I had so much fun making sushi rolls in my first book, *Vegan Lunch Box*. I included a long list of sushi fillings along with recipes for thick and thin sushi rolls, whole-grain rolls, and stuffed tofu pouches (*inari*). Where else can we go from there? Well, California Rolls are typically rolled inside out, so let's learn to do that! California Rolls are usually made with cucumber, avocado, and crab; seasoned carrots take the crab's place here.

Look for supplies and ingredients at Asian markets and some grocery and natural food stores.

Makes 3 to 4 servings

Special equipment you will need:
Bamboo rolling mat
    (available at Asian markets)

For the rolls:
1 recipe Sushi Carrots (page 183)
1 recipe Sushi Rice (page 154)
Sushi nori sheets (sheets of dry, toasted
    nori seaweed)
2 tablespoons toasted sesame seeds
2 tablespoons black sesame seeds (or more
    toasted sesame seeds, as desired)
Wasabi (optional)
1 English cucumber, peeled, seeded, and
    cut into strips
2 avocados, peeled and sliced

For serving:
Wasabi
Pickled ginger
Soy sauce

- Prepare the Sushi Carrots and Sushi Rice. Have your bamboo rolling mat, plastic wrap, and bowl of vinegared water ready (see Sushi Rice instructions).
- Cut a sheet of nori in half the short way. Lay one half-sheet lengthwise at the base of the bamboo rolling mat.
- Wet your hands with vinegared water and scoop up a ball of Sushi Rice (about the size of a large lemon). Spread the rice evenly over the nori, leaving a ½-inch strip at the bottom of the nori uncovered. Sprinkle the rice with toasted and black sesame seeds.
- Cover the top of the sushi with a piece of plastic wrap and flip it over (with strip of unriced nori still at the bottom).
- Lay your filling directly on the nori horizontally, an inch or so up from the bottom edge. Spread a pinch of wasabi across the nori first, if you like, then top with Sushi Carrots, cucumber strips, and avocado slices.
- Use your fingers to lightly moisten the top edge of nori with vinegared water; this will seal the nori roll. Immediately pick up the plastic wrap and begin rolling the sushi closed, wrapping the nori and rice around the fillings and pulling the plastic wrap off as you go. After it is rolled, bring the bamboo rolling mat up around it and press and squeeze on the mat to shape and firm up the roll.
- Unroll the mat, remove the plastic wrap, and place the sushi roll on a cutting board with the seam facing down. Cut the roll into six pieces with a very sharp knife, wiping the knife with a damp cloth in between cuts. Repeat with the remaining sushi rice and fillings.
- Serve your sushi with wasabi, pickled ginger, and soy sauce. Sushi should ideally be eaten the same day it is made.

Allergen Information ✳ Gluten-free, wheat-free, nut-free. Contains soy.

CHIK'N PAPRIKÁS

(Hungary)

Paprika is serious business in Hungary, where it is available in a range of heats from mild to hot. The sweet-hot flavor of paprika is essential in Hungarian cooking, as demonstrated in this vegan version of Hungarian Chicken Paprika.

Serve with white or brown rice, cooked barley, or Noodles with Poppy Seeds (page 147).

Makes 4 servings

2 tablespoons canola oil

½ medium onion, diced

1 pound (about a full tub) of chicken-style
   seitan, drained

1 green bell pepper, seeded and chopped

1 medium tomato, peeled and diced (page xiv)

1 tablespoon sweet or hot paprika

Salt and freshly ground black pepper, to taste

Vegan sour cream for serving

▸ Heat the oil in a nonstick or cast-iron skillet over medium-high heat. Add the onion and sauté, stirring frequently, until the onion is soft, about 8 minutes.

▸ Add the seitan, green pepper, tomato, paprika, and ½ cup water. Bring to a boil, lower the heat, and simmer, covered, for 15 minutes, until seitan is heated and the vegetables are cooked through.

▸ Season with salt and pepper and serve with vegan sour cream on the side.

Allergen Information ✳ Nut-free. Contains gluten, wheat, and soy.

CHIK'N POT PIE

Use small individual pie pans or mini-loaf pans to make pot pies that fit cozily into your lunch container.

<table>
<tr><td>

Makes 6 5-inch pies

</td><td>

1 pound (about a full tub) of chicken-style seitan, drained and cut into bite-size pieces

4–5 cups mixed steamed vegetables of your choice (potatoes, carrots, peas, cauliflower, green beans, onions, celery, etc.)

⅓ cup all-purpose flour

1 cup plain (unsweetened) nondairy milk

1½ cups vegan chicken-flavored broth or water

3 tablespoons nutritional yeast flakes

1 tablespoon low-sodium soy sauce

Salt and freshly ground black pepper, to taste

1 recipe Easy Piecrust (page 190)

</td></tr>
</table>

▶ Preheat the oven to 375°F.

▶ Place the diced seitan and vegetables in a large mixing bowl and set aside.

▶ Whisk the flour in a medium saucepan over medium-high heat for 2 minutes, until the flour smells toasty. Remove from the heat and whisk in the nondairy milk and chicken broth or water, along with the nutritional yeast and soy sauce. Return to the heat and whisk constantly until the mixture thickens and comes to a boil. Cook, whisking, for 2 minutes after it comes to a boil (this thickens the gravy and also cooks the flour so there is no "flour" taste to the gravy).

▶ Pour the gravy over the scitan and vegetables and stir to combine (if there are lumps of flour in the gravy, pour the gravy through a strainer). Check for salt and season with salt and pepper.

- Divide the filling between the pie pans and top each pan with pie crust. Crimp the edges closed and use a knife or small cookie cutter to cut a small hole in the center of each pie.
- Place the pies on a baking sheet and bake until the crust is cooked through and the mixture is bubbly, about 25 to 30 minutes.

Allergen ✳ Information — Nut-free. Contains gluten, wheat, and soy.

ENGLISH KIDNEY (BEAN) PIE

Traditionally this pie would be filled with steak and beef or veal kidneys. How much better it is when filled with vegetables and kidney *beans* instead!

Makes 4
5-inch pies

2 tablespoons olive oil

1 medium onion, diced

2 cloves garlic, minced

1 cup white button or cremini mushrooms, sliced

1 cup celery, cut in a large dice

1 cup carrots, peeled and cut in a large dice

1 (1-ounce) package beef-style vegetarian gravy mix

4 tablespoons vegetarian Worcestershire sauce

¼ teaspoon thyme

2 tablespoons fresh parsley, minced

1 (15-ounce) can kidney beans, rinsed and drained

½ pound (half a package) vegan frozen
    puff pastry, thawed at room temperature
    for about 40 minutes, or 1 recipe Easy
    Piecrust (page 190)

▸ Preheat oven to 375°F.

▸ Heat the olive oil in a medium saucepan over medium-high heat.
Add the onion and cook, stirring, until soft and browning, about
7 minutes. Add the garlic and cook, stirring, for another few seconds, then add the mushrooms, celery, and carrots. Cook, stirring,
until the mushrooms have released their liquid and the vegetables
are tender, about 10 minutes.

▸ Add 1 cup water, turn heat to high, and bring to a boil. Lower the
heat and stir in the vegetarian gravy mix, Worcestershire sauce,
thyme, parsley, and kidney beans. Cook, stirring, until the gravy
thickens, about 1 minute.

▸ Divide the filling between four small pie pans. Roll out the puff
pastry and top each pie with a round of pastry, crimping the edges
closed and cutting two or three vents in the middle to let the
steam escape.

▸ Place the pies on a baking sheet. Bake for 25 minutes, or until the
crust is golden.

SHEPHERD'S PIE VARIATION: To make Shepherd's Pie, another savory pie from England and Scotland, simply top the pie with a layer
of firm mashed potatoes instead of piecrust; use a fork to make decorative lines in the top, and bake as above.

> Allergen ✳ Information   Nut-free. Contains soy,
> gluten and wheat.

FLAUTAS

(Mexico)

We are blessed to live in a part of the country with a large Hispanic population, meaning we have access to dozens of fantastic Mexican restaurants, bakeries, and stores. At a local Hispanic grocery store we can watch corn tortillas being made right before our eyes and then take them home to make crispy fried flautas.

Look for small corn tortillas, around 4½ inches in diameter, to make flautas that fit perfectly in a small lunch container.

> **Makes 15 flautas, to serve 3**

Canola oil for frying

15 small corn tortillas

1 (16-ounce) can refried beans (plain, black bean, or any flavor you like)

▶ Cover the bottom of a large cast-iron pan with a layer of canola oil and heat over medium-high heat. When the oil is hot, put in a small corn tortilla for 3 to 4 seconds, turning once, just long enough for the tortilla to soften without browning or crisping.

▶ Pat the tortilla dry on paper towels, then spread 1½ tablespoons of refried beans slightly off the center of the tortilla. Roll the tortilla up as tightly as you can, then lay it in the hot oil seam side down (so the seam will seal shut). Fry until golden, then turn and fry on the other side, about 40 seconds per side.

▶ Repeat with the remaining tortillas and beans, using more canola oil as needed. Serve the flautas with salsa for dipping.

> Allergen Information ✳ Gluten-free, wheat-free, soy-free, nut-free. Contains corn.

GOLDEN INDONESIAN TEMPEH

Tempeh is my very favorite soy food. Both my son and I are crazy about its distinctive flavor and chewy texture, especially prepared as it is here, with a sweet caramelizing glaze and spicy red chile.

Try several brands of tempeh before deciding if you like it or not; not all brands taste the same, and some are quite strong. Look for solid, firm cakes of quality tempeh that won't crumble when you slice or fry them.

Makes 4 servings

---
4 tablespoons plus 2 tablespoons canola oil, plus more as needed

1 pound tempeh (2 8-ounce packages), cut into 16 strips

Salt, to taste

½ cup low-sodium soy sauce

6 tablespoons brown sugar

1 large shallot, minced

1 hot red chile, seeded and minced, or to taste

2 medium tomatoes, peeled and diced (page xiv)

▶ Heat 4 tablespoons of canola oil in a large nonstick sauté pan or well-seasoned cast-iron skillet over medium-high heat. When the oil is hot, add the tempeh strips and fry until golden, about 4 minutes per side (if you have to fry the tempeh in batches and the oil in the pan runs low, add more oil as needed). Remove the fried tempeh from the pan and set on a paper towel to drain. Sprinkle with salt if desired.

▶ Meanwhile, mix the soy sauce, brown sugar, and 3 tablespoons of water together in a small bowl and set aside.

- Heat the remaining 2 tablespoons of canola oil in the pan over medium-high heat. When the oil is hot add the shallot and chile and cook, stirring, until shallot is soft, about 1 minute. Add the diced tomato and cook, stirring occasionally, until the tomato has softened and cooked down, about 3 to 4 more minutes.
- Add the soy sauce mixture to the pan. Stir well, then add the fried tempeh and toss to coat. When the mixture comes to a boil, reduce the heat to medium-low and simmer until the liquid has cooked down to a syrupy glaze, about 5 minutes.
- This tempeh is good served hot or cold (I especially like it served cold on top of a fresh green salad).

> Allergen ✳ Information   Gluten-free, wheat-free, nut-free. Contains soy.

HULI-HULI TOFU

Hawaii's own version of barbecue sauce, sweetened with pineapple.

Makes 4 servings

1 pound Chinese-style firm tofu

⅓ cup ketchup

⅓ cup low-sodium soy sauce

½ cup unsweetened pineapple juice

1 teaspoon ground ginger

½ teaspoon garlic powder

½ teaspoon onion powder

¼ teaspoon yellow mustard powder

¼ teaspoon liquid smoke flavoring

▸ Slice the tofu into 8 large slices and place in a single layer in a baking dish.

▸ Combine the rest of the ingredients and stir well. Pour the sauce over the tofu and marinate the tofu for at least 30 minutes or up to several hours.

▸ Heat a nonstick outdoor grill or grill pan. Brush the grill with oil and grill the tofu for 3 to 5 minutes on each side, until golden brown grill marks form.

QUICK AND EASY VARIATION: Hawaiian-style barbeque sauce can also be purchased in the condiments section at grocery stores. Substitute 1 jar store-bought Huli-Huli or Luau BBQ Sauce for the homemade sauce and proceed with the recipe.

Allergen Information ✳ Gluten-free, wheat-free, nut-free. Contains soy.

JOLLOF RICE

(Africa)

Jollof Rice is served in many West African countries, including Liberia, Nigeria, Senegal, and Gambia. I've replaced the traditional chicken in the dish with chicken-style seitan.

What is seitan? Also known as wheat gluten or wheat meat, seitan (pronounced SAY-tan) is a chewy food made from the protein of wheat after the starch has been washed away. It's a great stand-in for meat in traditional recipes and a nice vegan protein food (20 grams per serving!) in its own right. Look for tubs of chicken-style seitan in the refrigerated section next to the tofu (I use Westsoy brand).

Makes 4 servings

1 cup long-grain rice

3 cups chicken-style broth (I use vegan chicken-style bouillon dissolved in hot water)

3 tablespoons canola oil

1 pound (about a full tub) of chicken-style seitan, drained

½ medium onion, diced

1 green bell pepper, seeded and chopped

1 tablespoon fresh grated ginger

1 large tomato, peeled and diced (see page xiv)

6 tablespoons tomato paste

½ teaspoon thyme

⅛ to ¼ teaspoon cayenne (the larger amount makes this dish quite spicy)

¼ teaspoon freshly ground black pepper

1 cup frozen peas or mixed peas and carrots

Salt, to taste

▶ Place the rice and 1¾ cups chicken-style broth in a medium saucepan. Bring to a boil, reduce heat to low, and cover. Cook on low, covered, until rice is tender and all liquid has been absorbed, about 20 minutes.

▶ Meanwhile, heat 2 tablespoons of the oil in a large, deep-sided skillet (preferably nonstick or well-seasoned cast-iron) over medium-high heat. Add the chicken-style seitan and cook, turning once or twice with a spatula, until seitan is browned lightly, about 5 minutes. Move the seitan onto a plate and set it aside.

▶ Heat the remaining tablespoon of oil in the skillet and add the onion. Cook, stirring often, until onion is soft and starting to brown, about 5 minutes (adjust the heat down as necessary if the onion is browning too quickly). Add the green bell pepper and ginger. Sauté for one minute, stirring constantly, then add the diced tomato and tomato paste. Cook, stirring frequently, until the tomato has softened and started to dissolve into the mixture, about 5 minutes.

▶ Add the remaining 1¼ cups broth along with the thyme, cayenne, and black pepper. Stir to combine, then add the seitan and the frozen vegetables. Bring to a simmer and cook, stirring occasionally, until the seitan is heated and the vegetables are cooked through, about 5 minutes.

▶ To serve, place a large serving of rice in a bowl and top with the seitan mixture.

Allergen ✳ Information   Nut-free. Contains gluten, wheat, and soy.

KASHA KUPECHESKAYA

(Russia)

Crumbled firm tofu takes the place of hard-boiled eggs in this traditional Russian recipe. Look for whole buckwheat groats (also known as kasha, or buckwheat kernels) at health food stores, Eastern European import markets, and Jewish markets.

To save time, look for toasted buckwheat. If you can only find raw, toast the kernels at home in a dry cast-iron skillet over medium heat, stirring, for 5 to 10 minutes, before proceeding with the recipe below.

Makes 2 to 3 servings

1¾ cups vegetable broth

1 cup whole toasted buckwheat groats (kasha)

8 ounces (about ½ tub) Chinese-style firm tofu

3 tablespoons canola oil

½ teaspoon turmeric

Salt and freshly ground black pepper, to taste

2 medium onions, peeled and sliced

▸ Bring the vegetable broth to a boil in a medium saucepan over high heat. Stir in the buckwheat and return to a boil. Reduce the heat to low, cover, and cook for 20 minutes, until the grains are tender but not falling apart. Fluff the kasha with a fork and set aside.

▸ Meanwhile, finely crumble the tofu with your fingers. Heat 1 tablespoon of the oil in a nonstick or cast-iron skillet over medium heat. Add the turmeric and cook, stirring, for 10 seconds, then add the tofu, salt, and a pinch of pepper. Cook, stirring frequently, until the tofu is starting to brown, about 8 minutes.

- ▸ Add the tofu to the cooked kasha and set aside. Wipe the skillet clean, return to heat and add the remaining 2 tablespoons oil. When the oil is hot add the onions and cook, stirring occasionally, until the onions are soft and golden, about 25 to 30 minutes. Turn the heat down if necessary to cook the onions slowly and let them caramelize.
- ▸ Add the caramelized onions to buckwheat mixture and stir to combine. Taste and season with more salt and pepper if desired.

VARIATIONS: Serve this kasha with Vegenaise on the side for diners to mix in (a traditional Russian way to enjoy this dish). To make this dish soy-free, substitute 1 (15-ounce) can rinsed, drained red beans for the tofu, skipping the instructions for cooking the tofu with turmeric and adding the beans to the cooked kasha along with the onions.

Allergen ✳ Information   Gluten-free, wheat-free, optionally soy-free, nut-free.

MANGO NOODLES

This Thai-inspired one-dish meal has it all: noodles, tofu, vegetables, and even fruit, all sparkling with that complex sweet-sour-salty flavor that makes Asian dishes so compelling. The actual cooking time on this dish is just 15 minutes or so, making it a quick fix in the morning if you do the prep work the night before: place the prepared garlic, ginger, and red chile in one bowl, the bell pepper, snow peas, baby corn, and scallions in another bowl, and the tofu and soy-lime marinade in a third. Refrigerate, covered, and in the morning dice the mango while the noodles are cooking and proceed with the recipe.

For this dish, look for medium-size flat rice noodles that look like linguini. Rice noodles can be found in the Asian foods section of your grocery store or at an Asian market.

Makes 4 servings

---

3 tablespoons low-sodium soy sauce

2 tablespoons freshly squeezed lime juice

2 teaspoons toasted sesame oil

2 teaspoons sugar

8 ounces (about ½ tub) Chinese-style firm tofu, cut into bite-size pieces

6 ounces flat rice stick noodles

2 tablespoons canola oil

1 tablespoon grated fresh ginger

2 cloves garlic, minced

1 fresh red chile, seeded and sliced

1 yellow, red, or orange bell pepper, seeded and cut into strips

6 ounces fresh snow peas

1 (15-ounce) can whole baby corn, drained and rinsed (about 1 cup)

5 scallions, sliced (both white and the
first inch of green)
1 fresh ripe mango, peeled and diced

▸ Stir the soy sauce, lime juice, sesame oil, and sugar together in a small bowl, then pour over the tofu and set aside to marinate while you prepare the rest of the dish.

▸ To cook the rice noodles, bring a large pot of water to a boil. Remove from heat and add the noodles to the hot water. Soak the noodles, stirring occasionally with a fork to keep the noodles from sticking together, until the noodles are soft but al dente, about 7 minutes (or according to package directions). Drain the noodles immediately and rinse under cold water. Set aside.

▸ Heat the canola oil in a skillet or wok over medium-high heat. Add the ginger, garlic, and red chile and cook, stirring, for 1 minute or until fragrant. Add the bell pepper, snow peas, baby corn, and scallions and stir-fry for 2 to 3 minutes, until the snow peas are bright green.

▸ Add the noodles and tofu to the skillet along with the lime juice mixture and cook, stirring, until the noodles are warmed through. Top with the diced mango and serve.

Allergen ✳ Information   Gluten-free, wheat-free, nut-free. Contains soy and corn.

MINI VEGGIE BURGERS

These homemade bean burgers are small enough that two or three can fit into your lunch box. Tuck them into Mini Burger Buns (page 196) with lettuce, tomato, and all the fixin's.

This recipe features my very favorite grain: amaranth. Amaranth is a tiny, gluten-free grain that is rich in protein and has twice as much iron as wheat. I love its flavor and sticky texture.

Makes 12 to 13
mini burgers

2 cups cooked drained lentils (see cooking instructions below or use canned)

½ cup dry amaranth

1 tablespoon olive oil

½ cup onion, finely diced (about half a medium onion)

1 large carrot, peeled and grated

¼ teaspoon celery seeds

½ cup quick or instant oats (or old-fashioned oats pulsed in a food processor)

2 tablespoons ketchup

2 tablespoons nutritional yeast flakes

½ teaspoon salt, or to taste

½ cup toasted sunflower seeds

▸ To cook the lentils, add 1 cup dry lentils to 3 cups boiling water and cook until the lentils are soft, about 30 minutes. Drain, measure out 2 cups of lentils and place them in a large mixing bowl (save any extra lentils for another use).

▸ To cook the amaranth, add the amaranth to 1 cup boiling water. Lower the heat and cook, covered, until the amaranth is cooked and all the water is absorbed, about 25 minutes. Add the cooked amaranth to the mixing bowl.

- Preheat the oven to 350°F. Line a baking pan with parchment paper and spray with nonstick spray. Set aside.
- Heat the olive oil in a nonstick or cast-iron skillet over medium heat and sauté the onion, carrot, and celery seeds until the carrot is soft, about 8 minutes. Add to the mixing bowl along with the oats, ketchup, nutritional yeast flakes, and salt.
- Grind the sunflower seeds into a coarse meal using a food processor. Add them to the mixing bowl and mix and mash everything together. Form mixture into 12 to 13 small patties, about 2¾ inches in diameter and ½ inch thick, and place them on the prepared baking sheet. Moisten your fingers with a bit of water to keep the mixture from sticking as you work.
- Bake for 20 minutes, until dry on the top, then flip the patties over and bake for another 10 minutes, until firm and brown.
- Serve immediately or let cool completely before packing. (Mini Veggie Burgers also freeze well.)

Allergen ✳ Information   Gluten-free (if using certified gluten-free oats), wheat-free, soy-free, nut-free.

MUJADDARA

(Middle East)

You won't believe how wonderful a simple dish of rice and lentils can be. Don't skimp on the oil or the onions.

Makes 4 servings

6 tablespoons olive oil

2 large onions, sliced

1¼ cups red lentils, washed and drained

1 cup white long-grain rice, washed
   and drained

1 teaspoon ground cumin

Salt and freshly ground black pepper,
   to taste

▸ Heat the oil in a large skillet over medium-high heat. Add the onions and cook, stirring frequently, until the onions are brown, about 20 to 25 minutes (turn the heat down as necessary if the onions are cooking too quickly).

▸ Remove the onions from the oil with a slotted spoon and drain on paper towels.

▸ Add the red lentils and rice to the oil along with the cumin. Sauté the rice and lentils, stirring gently, for 5 minutes. Add 3 cups of water. Turn heat to high and bring to a boil, then reduce the heat to low. Cook, covered, until the rice is done, about 20 minutes. Let stand off the heat, covered, for another 5 minutes.

▸ Fluff up the rice and lentils with a fork, season with salt and pepper, and top with the cooked onions.

VARIATION: Traditional Mujaddara calls for regular green or brown lentils, but I like the way red lentils (hulled lentils) cook quickly and disappear into the dish. If you would like to use green or brown lentils instead, soak them in water to cover for about 4 hours beforehand, then proceed with the recipe.

> Allergen ✳ Information   Gluten-free, wheat-free, soy-free, nut-free.

PUPUSAS

(El Salvador)

These are a little tricky if you've never worked with masa before, but hang in there. Pupusas look like small, thick tortillas; inside is a filling of refried beans. Pack them in your lunch with a small container of tomato sauce and a serving of Curtido (page 81).

Look for bags of masa harina (a special cornmeal used for making tortillas) at Hispanic groceries and in the Hispanic section of the grocery store.

Makes 6 pupusas

2 cups masa harina
1 cup refried beans, any flavor
½ cup fresh cilantro, chopped
Canola oil

▸ In a mixing bowl, mix together the masa harina and 2 cups warm water. Stir and knead together to form a moist, cohesive dough. The dough should be soft but not sticky; add more water a spoonful at a time if needed (the dough should not crack around the edges when you press it between your palms).

▸ Place ½ cup of the masa dough in your hand. Make a ball with the dough. Insert your thumb in the ball and make a hole in the center. Fill that hole with a large spoonful of the refried beans and about 1 teaspoon cilantro. Work the edges of masa up to cover the filling, then flatten the pupusa by clapping your hands together carefully to form a thick circle about 4 inches wide.

▸ Repeat with the remaining masa and refried beans.

▸ Heat a griddle or cast-iron skillet over medium heat and brush lightly with oil. Cook the pupusas on the hot griddle for about 4 minutes per side, until the surface is lightly browned and no longer sticky and the pupusas feel solid to the touch.

▸ Serve the pupusas topped with tomato sauce and Curtido (page 81).

Allergen ✳ Information   Gluten-free, wheat-free, soy-free, nut-free. Contains corn.

STUFFED EGGPLANTS

(Turkey)

Use small eggplants for this dish.

Makes 3 servings

6 small eggplants (approximately 4 ounces
each, 3 inches long)

2 tablespoons olive oil, plus more for
coating the eggplants

½ medium onion, peeled and diced

½ cup long-grain white rice

2 tomatoes, peeled and diced (see page xiv)

Salt and freshly ground pepper, to taste

1 tablespoon freshly squeezed lemon juice

1 tablespoon fresh parsley, chopped

▸ Preheat oven to 350°F. Trim the green tops off the eggplants. Rub each eggplant with olive oil and place in a baking dish. Cover the dish with a lid or with foil and bake the eggplants until soft to the touch, about 50–60 minutes.

▸ When eggplants are cool enough to touch, carefully cut a slit down the side, leaving the top and bottom intact. Push the eggplant open and use a knife and spoon (or melon baller) to scoop out part of the eggplant flesh to create a small cavity for stuffing. Chop all the eggplant flesh you have scooped out and set it aside.

▸ Heat the oil in a medium saucepan over medium-high heat. Add the onion and sauté until soft, about 5 minutes. Add the rice, stir to coat with oil, then add ½ cup water, the tomatoes, the reserved eggplant flesh, and salt and pepper. Bring to a boil, turn heat to low, and simmer, covered, until liquid is absorbed and rice is cooked, about 15 minutes. Stir in the lemon juice and parsley and taste for salt.

▸ Stuff each little eggplant with as much rice filling as it will hold (save any extra filling to stuff peppers or tomatoes . . . or do what I do and just eat it with a spoon!). Serve warm or cold.

┌───┐
│ Allergen ✳ Gluten-free, wheat-free,   │
│ Information   soy-free, nut-free.   │
└───┘

TOFU CHAR SUI

(China)

Char Sui is traditionally a dish of barbecued pork spareribs. For this recipe, you'll be using cubes of golden fried tofu instead. Look for them in packages in the refrigerated section at Asian grocery stores; the cubes are marked as "fried tofu" and are somewhat wrinkly and a deep golden brown on all sides. Fried tofu is deliciously chewy and "meaty," especially in this coating of sweet, savory sauce.

If you can't find deep-fried tofu where you live, substitute a pound of firm tofu that you have cubed and fried at home.

Makes 4 servings

⅓ cup sugar

⅓ cup low-sodium soy sauce

4 large cloves garlic, minced

2 teaspoons fresh ginger, grated

1 tablespoon toasted sesame oil

1 teaspoon Chinese five-spice powder

2 (8-ounce) packages 1-inch cubes of
    deep-fried tofu (about 50 cubes)

- ▸ Preheat oven to 450°F.
- ▸ In a mixing bowl, whisk together the sugar, soy sauce, garlic, ginger, sesame oil, five-spice powder, and 2 tablespoons water.
- ▸ Arrange the tofu in a 9 x 13-inch baking dish. Pour the sauce over the tofu and toss to coat. Spread the tofu in a single layer and bake until most of the sauce has been absorbed, about 20 minutes.
- ▸ These are great served warm or cold.

> Allergen ✳ Information — Gluten-free, wheat-free, nut-free. Contains soy.

TOFU TAMAGOYAKI

Tamagoyaki is a traditional Japanese egg omelet seasoned with sugar. Tamagoyaki is very common in Japanese bento boxes and sushi bars. The omelet is cooked in a special square pan, rolled up, sliced, and eaten cold.

In this recipe tofu takes the place of eggs. Use a sharp knife to cut the tofu tamagoyaki into square wedges or any shape you like for your bento box.

Makes 4 servings

2 teaspoons canola oil

1 (12.3-ounce) package firm silken tofu

2 tablespoons nondairy milk

1 tablespoon cornstarch

1 tablespoon sugar

¾ teaspoon salt

½ teaspoon turmeric

2 tablespoons all-purpose flour

- Preheat the oven to 350°F. Pour the canola oil into an 8 x 8-inch baking pan and put the pan in the oven as it warms up.
- Place the tofu, nondairy milk, cornstarch, sugar, salt, turmeric, and flour in a food processor fitted with the S blade. Process until very smooth, stopping to scrape down the sides as needed.
- Take the pan from the oven and tilt the pan around to spread the oil out to cover the entire bottom of the pan. Spread the tofu mixture out evenly in the pan with a spatula. Bake for 40 minutes, until completely set and golden on top.
- Cool completely on a wire rack. Remove the tamagoyaki from the pan with a thin spatula and invert it onto a cutting board. Cut the tamagoyaki into wedges with a sharp knife or pizza cutter. Refrigerate, covered, until ready to pack or eat.

Allergen ✳ Information — Nut-free. Contains gluten, wheat, soy, and corn.

TOFU TIGER

Here's an example of how bento lunches can be designed to look like cute characters or funny faces. This tofu is a tiger, but it could just as easily be a bear, frog, or kitten. Use your imagination!

Makes 1 tiger

Special equipment you will need:
Scissors
Animal head–shaped cookie cutter (optional)
Round paper punch (optional)
Toothpicks

1 pound Chinese firm-style tofu

Canola oil

Cooked Japanese rice for serving

Sheets of nori seaweed for decorating

Soy sauce for serving

▶ Cut a ¾-inch wide slice of tofu from the block (save the rest for another use). Use a sharp knife or a cookie cutter in the shape of a cat's head to cut the slab of tofu into a cat's head. (At this point it is helpful to use the container you plan to pack your lunch in as a guide to make your tofu tiger just the right size.)

▶ Heat a nonstick or well-seasoned cast-iron pan over medium-high heat. Drizzle the pan with enough oil to coat the bottom with a thin layer. When the oil is hot add the tofu and fry, without moving, until the bottom has turned golden, about 4 minutes. Flip the tofu over and repeat on the other side. Remove the fried tofu to a plate lined with paper towels and dab it dry.

▶ Fill your lunch container with a layer of rice and place the tofu on top. Use scissors and a sheet of nori to cut stripes and a face for your tiger (a round paper punch can be used to make the eyes and nose). Carefully dab the nori with a bit of water and immediately position the nori and pat it into place. Using toothpicks for this is helpful.

▶ Pack with a small container of soy sauce for serving.

Allergen ✳ Information — Gluten-free, wheat-free, nut-free. Contains soy.

ZARU SOBA

(Japan)

The taste of summer in Japan: a swirl of cold soba noodles being lifted with chopsticks, dunked in a dark, lusciously seasoned dipping broth, and brought to the lips. Refreshing and filling on a hot summer day!

Most soba noodles are a mixture of wheat and buckwheat flour. If you would like to make this dish gluten-free, Eden Foods makes 100% buckwheat soba (www.edenfoods.com).

Makes 6 servings

2 large whole dried shiitake mushrooms or
   ⅓ cup sliced dry shiitake
4 scallions, chopped (both white and
   part of green)
1 carrot, peeled and chopped
½ cup mung bean sprouts
1¼-inch slice of fresh ginger, chopped
1 clove garlic, chopped
1 2-inch piece of kombu seaweed
6 tablespoons low-sodium soy sauce
1 teaspoon sugar
6 tablespoons mirin (sweet Japanese
   cooking wine)
Pinch of shichimi togarashi (Japanese
   seven-spice blend; optional)
1 teaspoon toasted sesame oil
1 pound soba (Japanese buckwheat noodles)
½–1 sheet of nori seaweed, cut into fine
   shreds with scissors (optional)
Wasabi for serving (optional)
Chopped scallions for serving (optional)

- To make a stock for the dipping broth, combine the dried mushrooms, scallions, carrot, bean sprouts, ginger, garlic, and kombu in a medium saucepan along with 3½ cups water. Bring to a boil, reduce the heat to low, and simmer, covered, for 30 minutes. Strain the stock and measure out 2½ cups (save the rest to add to soups, cooking grains, etc.)

- Return the stock to the saucepan along with the soy sauce, sugar, and mirin. Bring to a boil, then lower the heat and simmer for 5 minutes. Add the shichimi togarashi (if using) and sesame oil. Let cool, then cover and refrigerate until completely cold.

- To make the noodles, prepare according to package instructions or as follows: bring a large saucepan filled with water to a rapid boil. Add the soba noodles. When the water returns to a boil, add 1 cup cold water. Repeat two more times. Keep simmering until the noodles are just tender, about 10 minutes. Drain the noodles and toss gently under cold running water until the noodles are cold. Drain.

- To serve, divide the soba noodles into serving dishes or lunch containers. Top each serving with fine shreds of nori, if desired, and pack or serve with a bowl of dipping broth. Diners can add a bit of wasabi or diced scallions to their dipping broth, if desired.

- To eat, take a bite of noodles onto your chopsticks, dip them into the broth, and enjoy.

Allergen Information ✳ Nut-free. Contains gluten, wheat, and soy (see note on gluten-free soba).

BEAN SIDES

ANASAZI BEANS

(Southwestern United States)

The anasazi bean is a beautiful white and brown mottled bean with an interesting history. The beans are thought to have been first raised and eaten by the Anasazi Indians, the famous "ancient ones," vanished cliff dwellers of the prehistoric Southwest. Dried anasazi beans were discovered in their ruins in New Mexico, sealed in an ancient clay pot over 1,500 years old. The bean has a mild flavor and is even said to contain less of the gas-causing carbohydrate that other beans possess.

The larger quantity of chiles will make this dish spicy. Use the smaller amount if you like it mild, or leave the chiles off altogether for the kids.

Makes 4 to 6 servings

2 cups dried anasazi beans

4 cloves garlic, peeled and minced

4 cups vegetable broth (in this recipe I like to use two vegetarian beef bouillon cubes dissolved in boiling water)

2 to 4 fresh green Anaheim chiles

1½ teaspoons salt, or to taste

▸ Soak the anasazi beans overnight in water to cover. Drain and rinse the beans, discarding the soaking liquid.

▸ Place the beans in a large saucepan with the garlic and vegetable broth. Bring to a boil, decrease the heat and simmer, covered, until the beans are tender, about 1 hour and 10 minutes.

▸ Meanwhile, preheat the oven to 450°F. Place the whole green chiles on a baking sheet and roast, turning often, for 30 minutes, or until soft, brown, and blistered. Immediately place the chiles on a plate and cover the plate with a large bowl, being sure that the bowl covers the edges of the plate and seals in the chiles. Let the chiles sit, covered, for 15 minutes.

▸ When the chiles are cool enough to handle, pull off the stems, remove the seeds and veins, and peel off the skin. Dice.

▸ When the beans are done, season with salt and sprinkle with the diced chiles.

QUICK AND EASY VARIATION: Instead of roasting your own chiles, use 1 (4-ounce) can roasted, diced green chiles, drained.

Allergen ✳ Information   Gluten-free, wheat-free, soy-free, nut-free.

BAKED FALAFEL

(Middle East)

Falafel are tasty little balls made from mashed chickpeas and spices. Usually the balls are fried, but I've baked them here instead. A little spritz of olive oil keeps the falafel from drying out during baking without adding much fat.

Makes 15 to 16 1-inch balls

Olive oil in a spray bottle, or nonstick olive oil cooking spray

1 (15-ounce) can chickpeas, rinsed and drained

2 tablespoons fresh parsley, minced

½ teaspoon onion powder

¼ teaspoon garlic powder

1 teaspoon ground coriander

1 teaspoon ground cumin

½ teaspoon salt

⅛ teaspoon cayenne

2 tablespoons whole wheat flour

3 tablespoons tahini (sesame seed paste)

▶ Preheat the oven to 350°F. Line a baking sheet with parchment paper and spray with olive oil spray. Set aside.

▶ Combine all the ingredients in a food processor fitted with the S blade and process until the mixture comes together in a coarse mash. Roll the mixture into 1-inch balls and set on the prepared baking sheet.

▶ Spray the tops of the falafel balls with the olive oil spray. Bake for 10 minutes, then turn the falafel over and bake for another 10 minutes, until lightly browned.

Allergen Information: Soy-free, nut-free. Contains gluten, wheat, and seeds.

BARBECUE BAKED BEANS

Kid Friendly

Start these beans in the slow cooker before you go to bed and you'll have perfect baked beans in the morning, ready to pack for lunch or carry on a picnic outing. Don't skip boiling the beans before placing them in the slow cooker; otherwise the acid in the tomato ketchup will stop the beans from ever getting tender.

Makes 8 servings

3 cups dry navy beans, soaked overnight
    in water to cover
1 small onion, diced
¾ cup ketchup
¼ cup maple syrup or Frugal Momma's
    "Maple" Syrup (page 60)
½ cup packed brown sugar
2 tablespoons prepared yellow mustard
1 tablespoon toasted sesame oil
¼ teaspoon liquid smoke flavoring
2 teaspoons salt, or to taste

▶ Drain the soaking navy beans and place them in a large saucepan with fresh water to cover. Bring to a boil, lower the heat, and simmer the beans until tender, about 30 to 40 minutes. Drain, reserving ¾ cup of the cooking liquid, and place the beans in a medium-size slow cooker. Stir in the diced onion.

▶ In a small bowl combine the reserved cooking liquid, ketchup, maple syrup, brown sugar, mustard, sesame oil, and liquid smoke flavoring. Pour over the beans and onions, stirring to mix.

- Cover and cook on low for 6 hours, stirring occasionally if possible. Mix in the salt.
- Serve warm or at room temperature.

Allergen ✳ Information — Gluten-free, wheat-free, soy-free, nut-free.

FRESH FAVA BEAN SALAD

(Turkey)

It's too bad that fresh fava beans are still hard to find in the United States. They are one of the many delights of Turkey, where they are eaten fresh with dill. Other regions in the Middle East also enjoy fava beans, both fresh and cooked dried. Fresh favas are a bit time-consuming to prepare, but once you've tried them, I'm sure you'll agree that they are worth the effort!

Makes 3 servings

3 pounds fresh fava bean pods
1 tablespoon olive oil
1½ teaspoons freshly squeezed lemon juice
¼ teaspoon salt, or to taste
1½ teaspoons fresh dill, minced, plus extra sprigs for garnish

- Preparing fresh fava beans is a two-part process. First, shell the beans, removing them from their furry outer pods. Hopefully you should have about 3 cups of beans.

- Place the beans in a saucepan, cover with water, and bring to a boil. Lower the heat and simmer for 10 minutes, or until the beans are tender when pierced with a knife. Remove from heat and immediately rinse well under cold running water until cool.
- Now here's the second part: you'll see that each fava bean has a thick outer skin. Use your fingers or a small knife to pinch a bit of the skin away and pop out the brilliant green beans underneath. Place the beans in a serving bowl and discard the skins.
- Mix the olive oil, lemon juice, and salt in a small bowl and pour the mixture over the fava beans. Sprinkle the minced fresh dill over the beans and garnish with a few extra sprigs of dill.

> Allergen ✳ Information   Gluten-free, wheat-free, soy-free, nut-free.

MUNG DAHL

(India)

Dahl (or dal) are simple dishes of cooked, seasoned legumes or pulses; they are quick-cooking, rich in protein, and easy to digest. Some form of dahl is cooked daily in most Indian homes and eaten with most meals.

Mung dahl are split, husked mung beans that are yellow in color. Look for them at health food stores, Indian grocery stores, and on-line. This dish can easily be made in advance and reheated; you will probably need to add more water while reheating, as it tends to thicken as it cools.

Makes 4 servings

2 tablespoons canola oil

1 medium onion, peeled and chopped

2 teaspoons fresh ginger, peeled and grated

1 jalapeño or other green chile, seeded
   and minced

1 cup mung dahl, rinsed in cold water
   and drained

½ teaspoon turmeric

⅛ teaspoon cayenne (optional, more or
   less to taste)

2 teaspoons freshly squeezed lemon juice

2 tablespoons fresh cilantro, chopped

Salt and freshly ground black pepper,
   to taste

▸ Heat the oil in a medium saucepan over medium heat. Add the onion and cook, stirring frequently, until the onion is soft, about 4 minutes. Add the ginger and jalapeño and cook, stirring, for another minute.

▸ Add 4 cups of water along with the mung dahl, turmeric, and optional cayenne. Raise heat and bring to a boil, lower the heat, and simmer, covered, until the mung dahl is fully cooked, about 30 minutes. Stir occasionally, especially toward the end of cooking, to keep the dahl from clumping or sticking to the bottom of the pan.

▸ Stir in the lemon juice, cilantro, and salt and pepper. Serve hot.

Allergen ✳ Information   Gluten-free, wheat-free, soy-free, nut-free.

PERFECT PINTO BEANS

(Southwestern United States/Mexico)

These creamy, smoky pinto beans are a perfect side dish for any Southwestern, Mexican, Central, or South American meal. Serve these simple beans as they are or garnish them with fresh salsa, diced onion, diced tomato, cilantro, or (my favorite) toasted pine nuts.

Toasted sesame oil and liquid smoke flavoring take the place of bacon in this recipe.

Makes 4 to 6 servings

2 cups dried pinto beans

4 cloves garlic, peeled and minced

1 jalapeño, sliced in half and seeded

1 tablespoon toasted sesame oil

¼ teaspoon liquid smoke flavoring

1½ teaspoons salt, or to taste

▸ Soak the pinto beans overnight in water to cover. Drain and rinse the beans, discarding the soaking liquid.

▸ Place the beans in a large saucepan with the garlic, jalapeño, sesame oil, liquid smoke flavoring, and 4 cups of water. Bring to a boil, decrease the heat and simmer gently, covered, until the beans are tender, about 50 minutes to 1 hour.

▸ When the beans are done, remove the jalapeño and add the salt.

Allergen Information ✳ Gluten-free, wheat-free, soy-free, nut-free.

CHAPTER 22

GRAIN SIDES

NOODLES WITH POPPY SEEDS

(Hungary)

Typically this dish would be made with wide egg noodles. Good vegan substitutes are ballerine/campanelle noodles, broken lasagna noodles, or any wide, ribbon-shaped noodles in short pieces.

Makes 4 servings	Salt, to taste
	½ pound noodles (see above)
	1½ tablespoons nonhydrogenated margarine
	2 tablespoons poppy seeds
	1 teaspoon sugar

▸ Bring a large saucepan of water to a boil. Add a sprinkle of salt and the noodles. Cook until the noodles are tender, about 11 minutes (or according to package directions).

▸ Drain the cooked noodles in a colander, rinse with cold water, and set aside. Return the saucepan to medium heat and add the margarine. Melt the margarine, then add the cooked noodles, poppy seeds, and sugar, and stir to combine. Heat, stirring occasionally, until the noodles are hot. Season with salt.

Allergen ✳ Information

Nut-free. Contains gluten, wheat, and soy.

ONIGIRI

Kid Friendly

(Japan)

In my first book I included a recipe similar to this one called Musubi. At the time I knew that these rice balls were also called *onigiri*, but I didn't understand the distinction. Thanks to *The Manga Cookbook*, I now know that *musubi* "primarily refers to the standard, triangle-shaped rice ball, whereas the word onigiri can be used for any kind of hand-packed rice ball."

The sky is the limit when decorating your onigiri with nori seaweed. I love to put happy faces on mine, using a happy face paper punch to punch out the nori. Or use scissors and come up with your own designs. A cute idea for little sports fans is decorating rice balls to look like soccer balls, footballs, and so on.

Makes 6 to 12 onigiri (depending on size)

Special equipment you may need:

Scissors (optional)

Rice molds (optional)

Paper punches (optional)

2 cups dry Japanese sticky rice

Salt (optional)

Nori seaweed, cut into strips or squares
   (optional)

- ▶ Cook the sticky rice according to package directions or as follows: rinse and drain the rice, then place it in a medium saucepan with 2½ cups water (1 part rice to 1¼ parts water). Bring to a boil and reduce the heat to low. Cover and cook on low for 25 minutes, until the water is absorbed and the rice is tender. Uncover and toss the rice with a rice paddle or wooden spoon, then allow to cool.
- ▶ Meanwhile, get a bowl of water ready.
- ▶ When the rice is cool enough to handle, moisten your hands with the water. Sprinkle a bit of salt onto your hands if you like. Spoon up a ball of rice, about the size of a golf ball. Use your hands to press the rice into a small ball, square, triangle, or other shape.
- ▶ If you have onigiri rice molds, you can use them instead of your hands to form the rice into shapes. Spray your mold with nonstick spray, then pack the rice in firmly.
- ▶ Once the onigiri have been shaped, you can cover all or part of the onigiri with nori seaweed, if you like. Use scissors or paper punches to cut sheets of nori into strips, squares, hearts, stars, or any other decorative shape. Use a bit of water on your fingertips to moisten the nori so it will stick, then place it on the onigiri.
- ▶ Cover the rice balls with plastic wrap until lunchtime. (Don't refrigerate, or the rice will get hard.)

VARIATION: Add a few drops of vegan food coloring to the cooked rice to make colored onigiri.

Allergen ✳ Information   Gluten-free, wheat-free, soy-free, nut-free.

ORANGE COUSCOUS

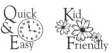

(Morocco)

Couscous is a staple food in the cultural area of North Africa known as the Maghreb, or West, which includes Morocco, Algeria, Libya, and Tunisia. It is usually served under a hearty stew, and although it looks like a grain, it is actually a very tiny semolina pasta!

Makes 6 servings

1 tablespoon olive oil

2 cups plain couscous

1½ cups orange juice

2 cups water

1 tablespoon agave or other honey substitute

1 teaspoon cinnamon

▸ Heat the olive oil in a saucepan over medium high heat. Add the couscous and stir constantly for 2 minutes, until couscous is fragrant and smells toasty. Add the orange juice and 2 cups water (the liquid will sizzle dramatically when it hits the pan) along with the agave and cinnamon. Stir to combine, then bring to a boil.

▸ Once the couscous comes to a vigorous boil, cover and remove from the heat. Let the couscous sit, covered, for 5 minutes.

▸ Uncover the couscous and fluff it well with a fork (fluffing separates the grains and keeps them from forming dense clumps). If the couscous is still a bit damp, cover again and let it sit for a few more minutes. Serve.

VARIATION: The version above is kept simple so it will go well underneath the more elaborate Moroccan Tagine (page 97). To turn this dish into a more flavorful stand-alone side dish (or excellent breakfast), add a handful of chopped dried apricots and raisins and ¼ teaspoon powdered ginger along with the liquid. Top with toasted slivered almonds just before serving.

Allergen 🌟 Information | Soy-free, nut-free. Contains gluten and wheat.

QUINOA VEGGIES

This is a colorful dish of quinoa and mixed vegetables. Quinoa can be found in the health food section of many grocery stores. Be sure to rinse the quinoa well under running water in a fine sieve before cooking; the grain coats itself with a natural insect repellent that tastes bitter if not removed.

Makes 6 servings

1 cup quinoa, rinsed and drained

2 cups vegetable broth or water

1 tablespoon olive oil

½ red onion, diced

2 stalks celery, diced

½ red, orange, or yellow bell pepper,
   seeded and diced

1 clove garlic, minced

2 medium zucchini, diced

½ cup frozen corn kernels

3 tablespoons fresh parsley, chopped

Salt and freshly ground black pepper,
   to taste

- Place the quinoa and vegetable broth in a small saucepan and bring to a boil over high heat. Turn the heat to low and cook, covered, for 20 minutes or until liquid has been absorbed. Fluff with a fork and set aside.
- Meanwhile, heat the olive oil in a medium saucepan or high-sided skillet over medium-high heat. Add the onion, celery, and bell pepper, and cook, stirring, until the onion is just soft, about 2 to 3 minutes. Add the garlic and stir for another 30 seconds, then add the zucchini and corn. Cook, stirring frequently, until the zucchini is crisp-tender, about 3 minutes.
- Add the cooked quinoa and stir well. Toss with the fresh parsley and season with salt and pepper, to taste.
- Serve warm or cold.

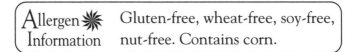

Allergen Information ✳ Gluten-free, wheat-free, soy-free, nut-free. Contains corn.

RICE WITH TOASTED MILLET

(Korea)

Toasting the millet before cooking gives this dish a nutty flavor.

Makes 2 to 3 servings	⅓ cup millet
	¾ cup short-grained rice, rinsed and drained

▸ Heat a dry cast-iron skillet over medium heat. Add the millet and cook, stirring, until the millet is toasted and fragrant, about 3 minutes.

▸ Place the rice and millet in a medium saucepan along with 1½ cups water. Bring to a boil, then give the rice a stir, turn the heat to low, and cook, covered, for 20 minutes. Remove the pan from the heat and let it sit, still covered, for another 15 minutes.

VARIATION: Substitute short-grained brown rice for the white rice and lengthen the cooking time accordingly. The millet will be softer but still tasty.

Allergen ✳ Information   Gluten-free, wheat-free, soy-free, nut-free.

SUSHI RICE

Kid
Friendly

(Japan)

Once you've mastered this recipe, you'll find sushi rice easy, delicious, and quite addictive. Sushi rice can be made into rolls, stuffed into tofu pouches, rolled into bite-size balls (perfect for toddlers), or made into "scattered sushi" (*chirashizushi*): arrange a serving of sushi rice in a bento or bowl and top with your favorite sushi fillings (tofu, blanched snow peas and asparagus, strips of nori, etc.).

Look for supplies and ingredients at Asian markets and some grocery and natural food stores.

Makes 3 to 4 servings

Special equipment you will need:

Wide, shallow wooden bowl or *hangiri* for
   mixing the rice

Wooden rice paddle or wooden spoon

Fan (electric or handheld)

2 cups uncooked sushi rice (short-grain
   sticky rice)

3 tablespoons brown rice vinegar

3 tablespoons mirin (sweet Japanese
   cooking wine)

3 tablespoons sugar

1 tablespoon coarse sea salt or kosher salt

▸ Rinse the rice several times in cold water until water runs clear. Put rice in a medium pot and cover with water. Let soak for 30 minutes.

▸ Drain the water, then add 2 cups fresh water (a ratio of 1 cup dry rice to 1⅓ cups water). Bring water to a boil, reduce heat, and simmer, covered, for 20 minutes (or use a rice cooker if you have one).

- Remove from heat and let sit, still covered, for 10 minutes. The resulting rice should be sticky, slightly wet, and shiny.
- While the rice is cooking, make the vinegar dressing by stirring together the vinegar, mirin, sugar, and salt until the sugar dissolves. (Note: don't use metal utensils when making sushi vinegar and sushi rice; the vinegar may react with the metal and create a disturbing taste.)
- Fill another small bowl with 1 cup water and 2 tablespoons vinegar. This vinegared water is used to wet the mixing tub and moisten your fingers to prevent the rice from sticking while you roll the sushi.
- Wet a large, shallow wooden bowl or special Japanese hangiri (wooden mixing tub) with water and pour off excess. Wet the tub a second time with some of the vinegared water and wipe off any excess.
- When the rice is done, heap the cooked rice in the center of the damp tub. Pour the vinegar dressing over the peak of the mound of rice. With a rice paddle or wooden spoon, cut through the mound of rice; toss with horizontal, cutting strokes. At the same time, use a fan to cool the rice as you toss. If you're coordinated, you can toss with one hand and fan with the other, but I find an electric desktop fan works well. Cooling and tossing in this way gives the rice good flavor, texture, and gloss.
- Once the rice has cooled to room temperature, it is ready to use. If you are not using the rice immediately, cover with a damp cloth. Do not refrigerate sushi rice; if it becomes too cold, it hardens.

Allergen ❋ Information — Gluten-free, wheat-free, soy-free, nut-free.

YELLOW COCONUT RICE

Quick
&
Easy

(Indonesia)

In Indonesia this rice is prepared and shaped into a cone for festivals and special occasions. The color yellow represents royalty, and the shape is meant to invoke the sacred mountain Meru.

Makes 4 servings

Two 4- to 6-inch stalks lemongrass, trimmed
2 teaspoons turmeric
¾ cup vegan chicken-flavored broth or water
1½ cups raw long-grain white rice, rinsed
    well and drained
1½ cups light or regular coconut milk
1 teaspoon salt, or to taste
1 red Chile Blossom (page 70) for garnishing,
    optional

▸ Cut the lemongrass stalks into 2-inch pieces and smash them with a kitchen pounder or the flat side of a heavy knife, just enough to bruise the lemongrass and release its aromatic oils without breaking it apart.

▸ Mix the turmeric with the broth or water. Put the rice, turmeric water, coconut milk, lemongrass, and salt in a medium saucepan and stir to combine. Bring to a boil over high heat, then turn the heat to low and cook, covered, 20 minutes or until rice is tender and all the liquid is absorbed.

▸ Before serving, remove the lemongrass pieces. Taste and add salt if needed. If you like, press the rice into a cone shape and garnish with a red chili blossom before serving or packing.

Allergen 🞷 Gluten-free, wheat-free,
Information   soy-free, nut-free.

CHAPTER 23

VEGETABLE SIDES

AFRICAN GREENS

(Africa)

An amazing array of healthy, nutrient-dense cooked greens are featured in African cuisine. Many of these African greens—bitterleaf, calalu, koko, kontomire, njamma-jamma, and okazi, to name just a few—aren't familiar or readily available to us here in the United States. That's okay, though, because in this recipe I use one that is: collard greens. Big bunches of large, smooth-leafed collard greens are found at farmers' markets and grocery stores throughout the United States, especially in the South.

The addition of peanut butter to these greens is very authentically African. Peanut butter (called groundnut in Africa) adds a rich quality to many African soups, stews, and vegetables and increases the amount of protein in the dishes as well. I highly recommend it. However, I am sensitive to the fact that many school districts are now asking that peanuts and other nuts never be brought to school due to serious allergy concerns. I couldn't in good conscience leave it out, but I have listed an allergen-free option at the end.

Makes 4 servings	1 large bunch of collard greens, hard stems removed, shredded (about 8 cups)
	3 tablespoons natural, smooth-style peanut butter
	1 teaspoon canola oil
	2 tablespoons diced onion
	1 small tomato, peeled and diced (about ½ cup) (page xiv)
	Salt, to taste

▸ Place the collard greens in a large saucepan and add enough water to almost cover, about 3 cups. Bring to a boil, reduce the heat to a simmer, and cook, covered, until the greens are just tender, about 5 to 7 minutes. Drain the greens over a bowl, reserving the cooking liquid. Set the greens aside.

▸ In a small bowl, mix together the peanut butter and ½ cup of the reserved cooking liquid. Stir to combine, then set the peanut butter mixture aside and return the saucepan to the heat.

▸ Heat the canola oil in the saucepan and add the onion. Cook, stirring often, until the onion is soft and starting to brown, about 3 minutes. Add the tomato and cook, stirring often, for another minute.

▸ Add the collard greens and the peanut butter mixture to the pan. Cook, stirring, until some of the liquid has cooked away and the greens are coated with a creamy peanut butter sauce. Season with salt.

ALLERGEN-FREE VARIATION: For a peanut-free variation, add the collard greens to the cooked onion and tomato and stir to combine. Season with salt, and serve.

Allergen ✳ Information   Gluten-free, wheat-free, soy-free, optionally nut-free.

ALL-STAR CORN

Cold cooked corn-on-the-cob is one of my son's favorite snacks; I wrap the corncobs individually in plastic wrap and keep them in the refrigerator so he can pull one out to eat whenever he wants.

This is a simple way to dress up sections of plain corn-on-the-cob for the lunch box. Use other cookie cutter shapes (flowers and hearts are nice) if desired.

Makes 1 serving

Special equipment you will need:
2 small graduated star-shaped vegetable or
   cookie cutters

1 cooked ear of corn (fresh or frozen)
1 large raw cucumber
1 large raw carrot

▸ Use a sharp, heavy knife to cut the corn into 2-inch pieces.

▸ Cut the cucumber into thin slices and use a star-shaped cutter to cut out star shapes. Place a cucumber star on top of each corn slice.

▸ Cut the carrot into thin slices and use a slightly smaller star-shaped cutter to cut out star shapes. Place one on top of each cucumber star.

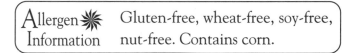

Allergen Information — Gluten-free, wheat-free, soy-free, nut-free. Contains corn.

ALOHA SWEET POTATOES

Sweet potatoes with butter, brown sugar, and coconut are a common sight at many Hawaiian luaus. I have toned down the fat and gotten rid of the sugar in this recipe, so the natural sweetness of the sweet potatoes shines through and the dish becomes a healthy side dish rather than—let's just admit it—a predessert dessert. A sprinkle of coconut invokes the original dish.

Makes 4 servings

¼ cup sweet flake coconut, raw or toasted

2 medium sweet potatoes

2 medium red garnet yams

4 tablespoons canola oil or melted
  nonhydrogenated margarine

Pinch of salt, or to taste

▶ To toast coconut, preheat the oven to 350°F, spread the coconut out in a thin layer on a baking sheet, and toast, stirring or shaking the pan occasionally, until the coconut is golden, about 5 minutes.

▶ Preheat oven to 400°F.

▶ Peel and dice the sweet potatoes and red garnet yams into ½-inch cubes. Toss with the oil or melted margarine and a sprinkle of salt, if desired, and spread in a single layer on a baking sheet.

▶ Roast, turning with a spatula two or three times, until the sweet potatoes are fork-tender and starting to brown, about 20 to 25 minutes.

▶ Let cool, then sprinkle with shredded coconut.

Allergen ✳ Information   Gluten-free, wheat-free, soy-free, nut-free.

ASIAN PORTOBELLOS

This is by far my favorite way to make portobello mushrooms. Use them in Vietnamese Salad Rolls (page 91) or serve them over rice with steamed baby bok choy and broccolini.

Makes 4 servings

1 tablespoon canola oil plus extra for the pan

3 cloves garlic, minced

1 tablespoon fresh ginger, grated

1 teaspoon Chinese five-spice powder

¼ teaspoon ground coriander

4 tablespoons mirin (sweet Japanese cooking wine)

2 tablespoons low-sodium soy sauce

2 tablespoons freshly squeezed orange juice

1 tablespoon toasted sesame oil

4 medium portobello mushrooms, rinsed clean and patted dry, stems removed

▸ Preheat the oven to 450°F. Brush a 9 x 13-inch baking dish with oil and set aside.

▸ Heat the canola oil in a small saucepan over medium heat. Add the garlic, ginger, five-spice powder, and coriander. Cook for 1 to 2 minutes, stirring constantly, until soft and fragrant. Remove from heat and add the mirin, soy sauce, and orange juice, and sesame oil.

▸ Arrange the portobello mushrooms gill-side up in a single layer in the prepared pan. Pour the marinade evenly over the mushrooms. Roast until the mushrooms are tender, about 20 to 25 minutes.

Allergen ✳ Information Gluten-free, wheat-free, nut-free. Contains soy.

BABY SQUASH MEDLEY

My son was disappointed when he bit into his first baby squash. "It just tastes like squash!" he complained. He was expecting squash babies to have a unique baby flavor.

Makes 4 servings

2 pounds baby pattypan squash

Bragg's Liquid Aminos or low-sodium soy
sauce in a spray bottle, to taste

2 tablespoons dry roasted pumpkin seeds

2 tablespoons dry roasted sunflower seeds

▸ Steam the whole baby pattypan squash until barely tender, about 5 to 10 minutes, depending on the size.

▸ Place the squash in a serving bowl, spritz with liquid aminos, and sprinkle with the pumpkin and sunflower seeds.

Allergen ✳ Information   Gluten-free, wheat-free, nut-free. Contains soy, seeds.

CARAMELIZED SQUASH
AND APPLES

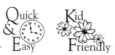

An excellent side dish for autumn, when winter squash and apples are at their best.

Makes 4 to 6
servings

----
1 small butternut squash

2 medium apples

3 tablespoons nonhydrogenated margarine

2 tablespoons brown sugar

Salt and freshly ground black pepper,
    to taste

▸ Preheat the oven to 400°F.

▸ Peel and seed the butternut squash and apples and cut them into ½-inch cubes. Place them together in a large mixing bowl.

▸ Melt the margarine and combine with the brown sugar. Drizzle over the squash and apples and toss to coat. Spread the squash mixture out on a baking sheet and season with salt and pepper.

▸ Roast, turning once or twice, for about 20 minutes or until tender and starting to brown. Season with salt and pepper.

Allergen ❋ Gluten-free, wheat-free,
Information   nut-free. Contains soy.

COLCANNON

(Scotland)

Colcannon is the only way I've ever gotten my son to (knowingly) eat kale. One night at dinner he kept shooting glances in the direction of my colcannon as he ate his pasta. Finally I asked, "Would you like some?"

"NO!" he shouted, then thought for a minute and shrugged. "Oh, okay." I put a small scoop on his plate, added a special little touch of salt, and sat back. He ate a small bite, then another, and another, and soon was asking for a bigger helping. He ate most of the colcannon himself, then finally remarked, "Well, mom, I guess you finally found a way to feed me kale." Hooray for colcannon!

Makes 4 servings

1 bunch kale, stems removed, chopped fine

4 medium russet (baking) potatoes, peeled
    and chopped

Plain (unsweetened) nondairy milk

Onion salt, to taste

Salt and freshly ground black pepper,
    to taste

Nonhydrogenated margarine, to taste
    (optional)

▶ Place the chopped kale in a steamer basket and steam until completely tender, about 20 to 25 minutes. Drain off any excess moisture and set aside.

▶ Meanwhile, cook the potatoes in water to cover until tender. Drain. Mash the potatoes with enough nondairy milk to make them creamy. Add the steamed kale, onion salt, regular salt, and pepper. Top each serving with a pat of margarine, if you like.

VARIATIONS: Substitute chopped cooked green cabbage for the kale. Add sautéed onions to either version, if you like.

> Allergen ✳ Information — Gluten-free, wheat-free, soy-free (if not using the margarine), nut-free.

ESPINACAS CON GARBANZOS (SPINACH WITH CHICKPEAS)

(Spain)

The flavor of this Spanish spinach dish is not to be missed. Serve it as it is with chunks of fresh artisan-style bread or over rice for a healthy comfort-food meal.

Makes 4 servings

---
1 tablespoon olive oil

2 cloves garlic, minced

1 pound fresh spinach (2 large bunches), washed and trimmed, cut into strips if leaves are large

1 cup canned chickpeas, rinsed and drained

1 teaspoon ground cumin

½ teaspoon ground coriander

¾ teaspoon paprika

Pinch of cayenne

Salt, to taste

▸ Heat the oil in a large saucepan over medium heat. Add the garlic and cook, stirring, for just a few seconds. Immediately add the spinach and cook, stirring, until the spinach is wilted, about 2 minutes.

▸ Add the chickpeas along with all the spices and ¼ cup water. Simmer over medium-low heat, uncovered, stirring occasionally, until most of the liquid has boiled away, about 15 minutes. Season with salt.

▸ Serve warm or at room temperature.

Allergen ✳ Information   Gluten-free, wheat-free, soy-free, nut-free.

FRIED NOPALES

(Southwestern United States)

Nopales are the flat, green pads of the prickly pear cactus. When cooked they taste something like lemony green beans, with a slippery quality like okra. Nopales have been eaten by Native Americans for centuries and are popular today in Mexican cuisine. You can find them in Hispanic markets and, more and more often, in regular grocery stores. My local market sells them whole or in bags, conveniently de-prickled and diced.

To prepare whole nopale pads, use kitchen gloves or a towel to hold the pad carefully, then use a sharp knife to scrape away any spines. Pare away the green edge around the outside of the cactus pad and discard it. Now dice or slice the pad as desired.

Makes 4 servings

1 pound nopale cactus pads, washed,
   trimmed, and diced (about 3 cups)
1 tablespoon canola oil
2 fresh green jalapeños, seeded and diced
½ teaspoon chili powder
Salt, to taste

▸ Place the diced nopale in a medium saucepan and add water to cover. Bring to a boil and boil for 30 minutes or until tender. Drain the nopale and rinse under cold running water (this will help remove some of the okra-ish slime).

▸ Heat the oil in a cast-iron skillet or sauté pan. Add the jalapeños and cook, stirring, for 1 minute. Add the nopale, the chili powder, and salt and cook, stirring frequently, for 5 more minutes.

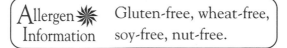 Allergen Information   Gluten-free, wheat-free, soy-free, nut-free.

HEAVENLY MUSHROOMS

Dry-skillet cooking is the secret to these heavenly mushrooms. Eat them as is or add them to cooked grains, soups, or casseroles. Use white button mushrooms, cremini, chanterelles, or any mushrooms you prefer.

Makes 4 servings

1 pound fresh mushrooms, cleaned, stems trimmed, quartered if large
2 tablespoons olive oil
2 cloves garlic, minced
2 tablespoons fresh flat-leaf parsley, minced
Salt, to taste

▸ Place the mushrooms in a large bowl filled with cold water. If the mushrooms are bobbing to the surface, rest a plate on top to hold them down. Soak the mushrooms for 10 minutes, then drain.

▸ Heat a large sauté pan over medium heat. Add the mushrooms and cover the pan with a snug-fitting lid. Cook, shaking the covered pan occasionally, until the mushrooms have released their liquid, about 20 minutes.

▸ Uncover (the bottom of the pan should now be filled with liquid), raise the heat, and cook until all the moisture has evaporated away. Reduce the heat back to medium and add the olive oil, garlic, and parsley. Cook, stirring frequently, for another 2 to 3 minutes, until the garlic is soft and the mushrooms are fragrant.

▸ Season the mushrooms generously with salt, to taste.

Allergen ✳ Information — Gluten-free, wheat-free, soy-free, nut-free.

INDONESIAN VEGETABLE PICKLES

(Indonesia)

Serve this simple vegetable side dish alongside rice and tempeh for an Indonesian-inspired meal. Shallots are small, brown-skinned members of the onion family and can usually be found near the garlic and onions in the produce aisle. Although they may be somewhat unfamiliar to us here in the States, they are used extensively in Indonesian cooking.

Makes 4 servings

1 large cucumber, peeled, seeded, and
    cut into matchsticks

1 medium carrot, peeled and cut into
    matchsticks

6 small shallots, peeled and cut into quarters

3 tablespoons white distilled vinegar

1 tablespoon sugar

1 teaspoon kosher salt

▸ Toss the cucumber, carrot, and shallots together in a bowl. Mix the vinegar, sugar, salt, and 1½ cups hot water together, stirring until the sugar dissolves. Pour over the vegetables, stir to combine, and refrigerate several hours or overnight.

Allergen Information — Gluten-free, wheat-free, soy-free, nut-free.

OVEN-ROASTED OKRA

Okra is a wonderful, nutrient-dense vegetable that hails from Africa. Roasting gives the okra phenomenal flavor, and leaving the okra pods whole lets you avoid the whole slime issue. Oven-Roasted Okra makes a great finger food in the lunch box.

When shopping for fresh okra, look for small, tender young pods. The older, larger pods can be woody and tough.

Makes 4 to 6 servings

2 pounds fresh okra, whole

2 tablespoons olive oil

2 teaspoons cumin

1 teaspoon freshly ground black pepper

Salt, to taste

▸ Preheat oven to 450°F.

▸ Rinse the whole okra and dry each pod with a kitchen towel (keeping them whole and as dry as possible helps minimize the slippery texture). Toss the okra with the olive oil, cumin, pepper, and salt.

▸ Arrange the okra pods in a single layer on a baking sheet and roast, turning occasionally, until the okra are tender and browned, about 15 minutes.

Allergen Information ✳ Gluten-free, wheat-free, soy-free, nut-free.

PALAK PANEER

(India)

Palak Paneer is a flavorful spinach dish, traditionally made with a soft white Indian cheese called *paneer*. Tofu is not commonly eaten in India, but in this dish tofu stands in quite handily for the *paneer*.

Makes 4 servings

1 teaspoon salt, plus more to taste

½ pound Chinese-style firm tofu, diced into ½-inch cubes

1 pound spinach (2 large bunches), washed and trimmed

1 tablespoon canola oil

½ medium red onion, diced

2 cloves garlic, minced, plus 1 clove garlic, minced

2 teaspoons fresh ginger, peeled and grated

1 teaspoon turmeric

½ teaspoon ground cumin

⅛ to ¼ teaspoon cayenne, or to taste

⅛ teaspoon nutmeg

1 tablespoon freshly squeezed lemon juice

2 tablespoons nonhydrogenated margarine

Salt, to taste

▶ Bring a medium saucepan filled with water to a boil. Add the salt and the tofu. Lower the heat and simmer gently for 5 minutes. Drain and set aside.

▶ Steam the spinach until tender, 3 to 5 minutes. Drain well and squeeze out any excess water, then chop the spinach on a cutting board.

- Meanwhile, heat the canola oil in a nonstick or well-seasoned cast-iron skillet over medium heat. Add the onion and cook, stirring frequently, until soft, about 4 minutes. Add the garlic and ginger and cook for another 2 to 3 minutes, then add the turmeric, cumin, and cayenne and cook, stirring, for 1 more minute (adjust the heat down as necessary if the onion and garlic are browning too quickly).
- Add the spinach and mix well. Lower the heat and cook, covered, for 5 minutes. Add the tofu cubes, remaining garlic, nutmeg, lemon juice, margarine, and salt. Simmer, covered, for another 10 minutes. Taste for salt, adding more if needed, and serve warm.

> Allergen ✳ Information — Gluten-free, wheat-free, nut-free. Contains soy.

PATATAS BRAVAS (FIERCE POTATOES)

(Spain)

Bravas means "fierce," referring to the fiery hint of Tabasco in this classic Spanish dish. Don't worry; you can tone down the Tabasco if you like your potatoes docile.

Makes 4 servings

4 tablespoons olive oil

4 medium russet potatoes (about 2 pounds), peeled and cut into ½-inch cubes

Salt and freshly ground black pepper, to taste

1 (8-ounce) can tomato sauce

1½ teaspoons prepared mustard
   (Dijon-style or any spicy, grainy mustard
   you prefer)
Several dashes of Tabasco sauce, more or
   less to taste

▸ Fill a saucepan or deep fryer with enough oil to submerge the potatoes (1½ to 2 inches or so). Heat the oil to 350°F (you will see the oil swirling and moving in the pot when it is hot enough). Adjust the heat as needed to maintain proper temperature; don't let the oil get too hot and start to smoke.

▸ Add the potatoes a few at a time and fry until golden brown on the outside and tender on the inside, about 8 to 10 minutes. Remove the potatoes with a slotted spoon and set on a paper towel to drain. Sprinkle with salt and pepper.

▸ Meanwhile, heat the tomato sauce in a small saucepan over medium-high heat. Cook, stirring, until warmed through and bubbling, about 3 minutes. Add the mustard and Tabasco and stir well.

▸ Just before serving, pour some sauce over each serving of potatoes (pack the tomato sauce and potatoes separately in the lunch box).

Allergen ✳ Information   Gluten-free, wheat-free, soy-free, nut-free.

POTATO PARSNIP LATKES

Latkes are a traditional Jewish dish. Although these fried potato cakes are usually eaten at Hanukkah time, they are delicious enough to eat all year long. Serve them with Applesauce (page 205) and/or vegan sour cream.

Makes 8 to 10 latkes

½ pound new potatoes, such as Yukon Gold

¾ teaspoon kosher salt

2 medium parsnips, peeled and grated

½ onion, grated

2 tablespoons chopped fresh chives

Freshly ground black pepper, to taste

3 tablespoons olive oil, plus more as needed

▸ Peel the potatoes and shred them using a food processor fitted with a large shredding disk or a hand grater with large holes. Place the shredded potatoes in a large mixing bowl, sprinkle them with salt, and toss to coat well. Let the potatoes sit for at least 5 minutes.

▸ Take large handfuls of the potatoes and squeeze out as much liquid as possible, transferring the potatoes to a clean mixing bowl as you go.

▸ Add the grated parsnip and onion to the potatoes along with the chives and a few grinds of pepper.

▸ Heat the olive oil in a large nonstick skillet or well-seasoned cast-iron skillet over medium heat. When the oil is hot (a strand of potato should sizzle when it hits the oil), pick up a handful of potato shreds, give them one last good squeeze, then drop into the oil. Repeat, making as many mounds as will fit in the pan without touching. Press the mounds flat with your spatula and tuck the edges in to maintain an even thickness.

- Adjust the temperature down as needed to maintain a sizzle (you don't want the latkes to brown too quickly). Cook until the bottom has turned a nice golden brown, about 8–10 minutes. Flip with a spatula and cook on the other side until golden brown, another 6–8 minutes. Drain on paper towels for a moment to remove excess oil.
- Repeat with the rest of the potato shreds, adding more oil to the pan as needed.

Allergen ✳ Information   Gluten-free, wheat-free, soy-free, nut-free.

RED CURRY VEGETABLES

(Thailand)

This is my favorite way to enjoy the amazing Asian long beans you find at farmers' markets and Asian grocery stores. Often well over a foot in length, these flexible green beans look like long green noodles. Look for thin, young long beans, which will be the most tender and cook the fastest. If you can't find long beans where you live, substitute regular green beans and adjust the cooking time as needed.

Jars of Thai red curry paste are available in the Asian section of the grocery store or at Asian import markets. Add more or less according to your taste. (I prefer one tablespoon, while my husband would use an entire jar at once.)

Feel free to substitute other vegetables as you see fit. Broccoli, bell peppers, or snow peas would not be amiss here.

Makes 4 servings

2 tablespoons canola oil

1 to 3 tablespoons Thai red curry paste
   (I use Thai Kitchen Red Curry Paste)

2 cups Asian long beans or green beans,
   cut into bite-size pieces

2 cups baby bok choy, cut into bite-size pieces
   (both leaves and stems)

2 tablespoons low-sodium soy sauce

1 tablespoon sugar

▶ Heat the oil in a skillet over medium heat. Add the red curry paste and cook, stirring, until the paste is fragrant, about 3 minutes.

▶ Add the beans and bok choy and stir-fry for 3 minutes, until the bok choy leaves are wilting and the beans are almost tender.

▶ Mix the soy sauce and sugar together and add to the skillet along with ½ cup water. Stir to combine and simmer, uncovered, until the beans are just tender, another 3 minutes or so (increase the cooking time if needed for thicker green beans, adding more water if the skillet gets dry).

▶ Serve hot or cold.

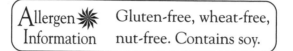

Allergen Information — Gluten-free, wheat-free, nut-free. Contains soy.

ROASTED VEGGIE KABOBS

These kabobs can also be cooked on an outdoor grill.

Makes 12 skewers
(4 servings)

Special equipment you will need:
12 small (6-inch) wooden or bamboo skewers

2 tablespoons olive oil
1 tablespoon freshly squeezed lemon juice
2 teaspoons white wine vinegar
1 clove garlic, minced
¼ teaspoon cumin
Salt and freshly ground black pepper, to taste
3–4 small zucchini, cut into ½-inch slices
14–16 whole cherry tomatoes
14–16 whole button mushrooms (white or cremini), washed and trimmed
1 red, orange, or yellow bell pepper, seeded and cut into ¾-inch squares

▸ Preheat the oven to 450°F.
▸ To make the marinade, whisk together the olive oil, lemon juice, vinegar, garlic, cumin, and salt and pepper.
▸ Alternate chunks of zucchini, cherry tomatoes, mushrooms, and bell pepper squares on the skewers (beginning and ending with squares of pepper or mushrooms helps hold everything together).
▸ Arrange the skewers in a single layer in a baking dish and pour the marinade evenly over the top.
▸ Roast the kabobs, turning once or twice, until the vegetables are tender, about 25 minutes.
▸ These are good served warm or cold.

Allergen ✳ Information Gluten-free, wheat-free, soy-free, nut-free.

STIR-FRIED ARAME WITH CARROTS AND GINGER

Kid Friendly

(Japan)

If you are new to eating sea vegetables (also known as seaweed), this dish is a great place to start. Arame is the mildest of the sea veggies, with an almost-sweet taste that pairs beautifully with carrots and fresh ginger. Even children love it; my two-year-old niece packed this dish away like nobody's business.

Arame, like other sea vegetables, is rich in minerals like calcium, iron, and iodine. It's quick and easy to prepare. Look for dried arame at health food stores or online at www.edenfoods.com.

Makes 4 servings

1 cup dried arame, loosely packed

1 tablespoon plus 2 teaspoons low-sodium soy sauce

1 tablespoon toasted sesame oil

2 medium carrots, peeled and coarsely grated (I use a food processor fitted with a grating blade)

1 tablespoon fresh ginger, peeled and sliced (cut into thin slices the same size as the grated carrot)

Toasted sesame seeds

▸ Rinse the arame, then place it in a small saucepan with water to cover. Add 1 tablespoon soy sauce and bring to a boil over high heat. Turn the heat to medium-low and simmer, slightly covered, for 15 minutes. Drain and set aside.

▸ Heat the sesame oil in a nonstick or well-seasoned cast-iron skillet or wok over medium-high heat. Add the carrots and ginger and stir-fry for 2 minutes. Add the arame and stir-fry for another 4 minutes, until the carrots are just tender. Add 2 teaspoons soy sauce, toss well, and cook for another few seconds, until the soy sauce has cooked away.

▸ Sprinkle with toasted sesame seeds. This dish is good served warm or cold.

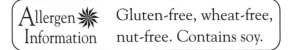

Allergen Information: Gluten-free, wheat-free, nut-free. Contains soy.

STIR-FRIED WATERCRESS

There are no words to express how much I love this dish. Watercress is a true nutritional powerhouse: by weight, it has more calcium than milk, more vitamin C than an orange, and more absorbable iron than spinach! Stir-frying watercress and tossing it with a simple Asian dressing eliminates the bitterness of the raw green and transforms it into something I could eat every day.

Makes 2 servings

2 teaspoons toasted sesame oil

2 large bunches watercress, washed and trimmed

1 teaspoon fresh ginger, grated

2 teaspoons low-sodium soy sauce

1 teaspoon rice vinegar

1 teaspoon toasted sesame seeds

▸ Heat the sesame oil in a nonstick wok or cast-iron skillet over high heat. Add the watercress and ginger and stir-fry until tender, about 3 minutes.

▸ Drain any excess liquid from the cooked watercress. Toss the watercress with the soy sauce and vinegar and sprinkle with sesame seeds. Serve warm or cold.

Allergen ✳ Information   Gluten-free, wheat-free, nut-free. Contains soy.

SWEET PEAS WITH MINT

(England)

Mint adds a refreshing taste to this simple pea dish.

Makes 4 to 6
servings

---

1 pound frozen green peas

¼ cup nonhydrogenated margarine

2 tablespoons fresh mint, minced

1 teaspoon sugar

Salt, to taste

▸ Cook the frozen peas in a medium saucepan according to package directions. Drain and set aside.

▸ Return the saucepan to the stove and add the margarine. Melt the margarine and add the mint and sugar. Stir to combine, then add the peas. Cook, stirring, until the peas are warmed through. Season with salt.

Allergen ✳ Information — Gluten-free, wheat-free, nut-free. Contains soy.

SUSHI CARROTS

Use these seasoned, cooked carrots as a filling for California Rolls (page 110).

Makes about 1 cup

---
2 medium carrots, peeled and cut into
    matchsticks
4 teaspoons sugar
2 teaspoons low-sodium soy sauce
1 1-inch piece kombu seaweed

▸ Combine all ingredients with ⅔ cup water in a small saucepan. Bring to a boil, reduce heat, and simmer over low heat until the carrot strips are tender but not falling apart, about 6 to 7 minutes. Drain the carrot strips and refrigerate until cool.

Allergen ✳ Information
Gluten-free, wheat-free, nut-free. Contains soy.

TERIYAKI GREEN BEANS

Kid Friendly

My son's favorite way to eat green beans. Small, tender green beans work best in this dish; look for ones marked "French green beans" at the grocery store.

Makes 4 servings

Salt

1 pound fresh whole green beans, washed and trimmed

1½ tablespoons toasted sesame oil

2 cloves garlic, minced

2 tablespoons low-sodium soy sauce

½ teaspoon sugar

Toasted sesame seeds

▸ Bring a medium saucepan filled with lightly salted water to a boil. Add the green beans and boil until they are crisp-tender, about 5 minutes (longer if the beans are large). Immediately drain the beans and plunge them into ice water or rinse them well with cold water to halt the cooking. Drain well.

▸ Heat the oil in a sauté pan or wok over medium-high heat. Add the garlic and stir for a few seconds, then add the green beans, soy sauce, and sugar and stir-fry until the beans are well-coated and warm, about 2 minutes.

▸ Sprinkle with toasted sesame seeds.

▸ These beans are delicious served warm or at room temperature.

Allergen Information ✳ Gluten-free, wheat-free, nut-free. Contains soy.

TRINIDAD SPINACH

(Trinidad)

There is a large Indian influence on much of the cooking of Trinidad, a small island off the coast of Central America, where hundreds of thousands of Indians came as indentured servants to work the sugar plantations. This spinach is one of their dishes, perfect alongside an Indian dahl and flatbread, or with a dish of beans and coconut rice.

Makes 4 servings

1 tablespoon canola oil
½ medium onion, diced
1 clove garlic, minced
½ small red or green chile, seeded and diced
1 pound fresh spinach, washed and cut into
    strips (2 large bunches)
Pinch of salt, or to taste

▸ Heat the oil in a large saucepan over medium heat. Add the onion and cook, stirring, until soft, about 5 minutes. Add the garlic and chile and cook, stirring, for another minute.

▸ Add the spinach and salt. Turn the heat to medium-low and cover the pan. Cook, stirring occasionally, until the spinach is soft and has released a lot of liquid, about 15 minutes.

▸ Uncover the pan, turn the heat to high, and cook until almost all the liquid has cooked away, about 5 minutes. Taste for salt and add more if desired.

Allergen ✳ Information   Gluten-free, wheat-free, soy-free, nut-free.

TZIMMES

Tzimmes is a traditional Ashkenazi Jewish dish served on Rosh Hashanah (Jewish New Year). "Tzimmes" is a Yiddish word that roughly translates as "mishmash" or "confusion." Perhaps those who named the dish were referring to the confusion of having vegetables and fruits together in one dish.

Makes 6 servings

1 pound carrots, peeled and sliced into
    ½-inch pieces
½ cup dried plums (prunes)
½ cup dried apricots
½ cup orange juice
1 3-inch cinnamon stick
2 2-inch long strips of orange zest
    (peeled from a fresh orange with a
    vegetable peeler)

▸ Place all ingredients in a medium saucepan along with ½ cup water. Bring to a boil, lower the heat, and simmer, covered, for 20 minutes. Remove the lid and simmer uncovered for another 10 minutes, or until carrots are tender and liquid is almost all absorbed.

▸ Remove the cinnamon stick and strips of orange zest before serving.

VARIATION: Substitute sliced sweet potato for some or all of the carrots.

Allergen Information ✳ Gluten-free, wheat-free, soy-free, nut-free.

BREADS AND MUFFINS

QUICK BREADS

BOSTON BROWN BREAD MUFFINS

(New England)

The early Colonial settlers in New England did not have ovens, so they devised a method to steam-cook their bread instead, making hearty loaves out of a mixture of cornmeal, rye, and wheat to stretch their scarce wheat supply. They sweetened the loaves with nutritious molasses. The resulting Boston Brown Bread was steam-cooked in a coffee can or round mold.

Instead of steaming, I decided to bake my Boston Brown Bread into muffins, making perfect individual servings for a lunch box. If you like, bake this batter in a round or regular loaf pan instead and increase the baking time to about 1 hour.

Makes 16 muffins

4 teaspoons apple cider vinegar

About 2 cups plain soymilk

1 cup finely ground cornmeal

1 cup whole rye flour

1 cup all-purpose flour

2 teaspoons baking soda

½ teaspoon kosher salt

⅔ cup firmly packed brown sugar

¼ cup blackstrap molasses

¾ cup raisins

½ cup chopped walnuts (optional)

▸ Preheat the oven to 350°F. Spray a muffin pan with nonstick cooking spray and set aside.

▸ Pour the vinegar into a 2-cup or larger liquid measuring cup. Fill the measuring cup with soymilk to the 2-cup level. Set aside (the mixture will curdle).

▸ In a large mixing bowl, whisk together the cornmeal, rye flour, white flour, baking soda, and salt. Add the brown sugar, molasses, and soymilk mixture and stir to combine. Fold in the raisins and walnuts.

▸ Spoon the batter into the prepared muffin pan. Bake for 15 to 17 minutes, until a toothpick or cake tester inserted into the center of a muffin comes out cleanly. Immediately remove the muffins from the pan and let cool on a wire rack. Store in an airtight container.

Allergen ✳ Information — Contains gluten, wheat, soy, and nuts (optional).

CORNCOB CORNBREAD

(Southwestern United States)

These little cornbread "sticks" are flecked with bits of fresh corn. Serve them alongside any soup, chili, or stew, or with margarine and jam for a simple dessert.

For this recipe you'll need a cast-iron cornstick baking pan. Look for them anywhere cast iron is sold. Or bake the batter in any size muffin pan you prefer, adjusting the cooking time as necessary.

Makes 15 4¾-inch long cornsticks or 12 regular muffins

⅓ cup maple syrup or Frugal Momma's "Maple" Syrup (page 60)

⅓ cup canola or corn oil

1⅓ cups plain nondairy milk

1 cup whole wheat pastry flour

1 cup finely ground cornmeal

1 tablespoon baking powder

1 teaspoon kosher salt

1 cup fresh or thawed frozen corn kernels

▸ Preheat the oven to 350°F. Brush the cast-iron cornstick pan with canola or corn oil and set it in the oven to preheat.

▸ In a small mixing bowl combine the maple syrup, canola oil, and nondairy milk. In another bowl whisk together the flour, corn-meal, baking powder, and salt.

▸ Mix the wet and dry ingredients together. Add the corn kernels and stir to combine.

▸ Fill the cornstick molds with batter to the top, filling in all the little nooks and crannies. Bake for 25 minutes, until a toothpick or cake tester comes out cleanly and the cornsticks are golden.

▸ Let the cornsticks cool 15 minutes in the pan before turning out.

Allergen ✳ Information   Soy-free, nut-free. Contains gluten, wheat, corn.

EASY PIE CRUST

I love wrapping savory fillings in flaky piecrust! This is the same simple piecrust recipe I used in my first book to make Spanish Empanadas, Cornish Pasties, Aloo Samosas, and more. This time around I've used it to make individual Chik'n Pot Pies (page 113) and English Kidney (Bean) Pies (page 114).

Makes 1 9-inch
pie shell

2 cups all-purpose flour (or half white,
   half whole wheat pastry flour)
1 teaspoon kosher salt
⅔ cup nonhydrogenated shortening
5 to 7 tablespoons ice water, as needed

▸ Have a cup of ice water and a tablespoon ready.
▸ Sift or whisk together the flour and salt in a mixing bowl. Dot the top of the flour mixture with tablespoons of the shortening. Cut the shortening into the flour with a pastry cutter, or cut the shortening into the flour by tossing and rubbing the flour and shortening together with your hands or fingers. Keep at it until the mixture resembles coarse meal, and all visible lumps of shortening are gone.
▸ Lightly drizzle in the water a tablespoon at a time, stirring with a wooden spoon or your fingers, until you can bring the dough together in a ball. Add a few extra drops if the dough is still crumbly. Shape the dough into a ball, then proceed with your recipe.
▸ If it's a hot day, you may wish to refrigerate the dough for 15 minutes before rolling and shaping.

Allergen ✳ Soy-free (if using soy-free shortening),
Information nut-free. Contains gluten and wheat.

PLOYES (BUCKWHEAT CRÊPES)

(Canada)

You'll find many recipes for ployes in eastern Canada and New England. These thin buckwheat griddle cakes are cooked on only one side, leaving open holes all over the top side—a distinguishing sign of a good ploye. Best of all, they are naturally vegan. Serve them with baked beans, maple syrup, molasses, or jam.

Makes 8 ployes

1 cup buckwheat flour
1 cup all-purpose flour
2 teaspoons baking powder
1 teaspoon salt

▶ Sift the buckwheat flour, white flour, baking powder, and salt together into a medium mixing bowl. Add 1½ cups cold water and whisk until smooth. Add ½ cup boiling water and stir to combine.

▶ Cover the bowl with plastic wrap and let the batter sit for 30 minutes. Toward the end of that time, begin heating a nonstick or well-seasoned cast-iron skillet or griddle over medium-high heat.

▶ Pour ⅓ cup batter onto the hot, ungreased skillet. (The batter should be the consistency of cake batter and should spread out on its own to form a thin, round ploye about 6 to 7 inches across. If it's too thick, add extra water to the mixing bowl and stir to combine.)

▶ Cook without turning until the bottom is crisp and the top is dry and dotted with large holes, about 2 minutes. Remove from the skillet and serve, or cool on a wire rack. Repeat with the remaining batter.

Allergen ✳ Information — Soy-free, nut-free. Contains gluten and wheat.

SOUR CREAM SCONES

These are simply the best scones. Serve them the next time you have guests over for breakfast or tea; no one will even guess they are vegan.

Makes 10 to 12 scones

¼ cup vegan sour cream

Zest of one orange (about ½ tablespoon)

¼ cup freshly squeezed orange juice

1¼ cups all-purpose flour

1½ teaspoons baking powder

½ teaspoon kosher salt

3 tablespoons sugar

3 tablespoons nonhydrogenated margarine, cold, cut into pieces

¼ cup dried currants

Nondairy milk and cinnamon-sugar for topping

▸ Preheat oven to 425°F. Line a baking sheet with parchment paper, spray with nonstick spray, and set aside.

▸ In a small mixing bowl, combine the vegan sour cream, orange zest, and orange juice. Set aside.

▸ Sift or whisk together the flour, baking powder, salt, and sugar. Cut in the margarine with a pastry cutter or your fingers, until the mixture resembles coarse meal and all visible lumps of margarine are gone. Stir in the sour cream mixture and the currants.

▸ Turn the dough out and press into a ¾-inch thick circle. Cut into 10 to 12 wedges with a large knife. Brush the tops with nondairy milk and sprinkle with cinnamon-sugar.

▸ Place the scones 2 inches apart on the baking sheet. Bake until golden, about 10 to 12 minutes. Cool on a wire rack.

Allergen ✳ Information | Nut-free. Contains gluten, wheat, and soy.

GRILLED VEGETABLE STROMBOLI

(Italy)

Typically, this Italian rolled sandwich is made with a filling of cheese and meat, but I like a filling of grilled eggplant and zucchini instead. Next time you pull out the grill for a vegan BBQ, you can throw on a few extra veggies and save them for stromboli.

Makes 4 servings

1 large eggplant

2 medium zucchini

Kosher salt as needed

Olive oil for grilling

1⅛ cups warm water (110°F)

1 tablespoon active dry yeast

Pinch of sugar

2 tablespoons olive oil

1 teaspoon kosher salt

2½ to 3 cups all-purpose flour or white bread flour

1 head of Roasted Garlic (see page 64)

Italian herb seasoning mix, to taste

Salt and freshly ground black pepper, to taste

½ teaspoon poppy seeds

▶ To make the vegetables, trim off the tops of the eggplant and zucchini, then slice them lengthwise into strips, cutting them as thinly as possible (a mandolin may be helpful here). Lay the strips out in a single layer and sprinkle both sides of them with salt. Let the strips sit for 30 minutes (this will help remove some of the moisture from the vegetables).

- ▸ Heat a nonstick grill or grill pan. Pat the vegetables dry and brush them lightly with olive oil. Grill, turning halfway, until the strips are soft and have brown grill marks. Set the vegetable strips aside to cool, or refrigerate until needed.
- ▸ To make the dough, place the warm water in a mixing bowl. Sprinkle the yeast and sugar into the warm water and stir well. Let the mixture sit for 5 minutes to dissolve the yeast.
- ▸ Add the olive oil, salt, and 2 cups of the flour. When the dough begins to form a ball, turn the dough out onto a lightly floured surface and knead. As you knead, add just enough of the remaining flour to keep the dough from sticking. Knead for about 10 to 15 minutes, until the dough is smooth, elastic, and supple.
- ▸ Place the dough in a well-oiled mixing bowl, turning to cover the top of the dough with some of the oil. Cover with plastic wrap and a kitchen towel, and place in a warm, draft-free place to rise until doubled in bulk, about 1 hour.
- ▸ Preheat the oven to 375°F. Line a baking sheet with parchment paper, spray with nonstick spray, and set aside.
- ▸ Turn the dough out onto a lightly floured surface and roll into a flat rectangle, about 10 x 12 inches.
- ▸ Squeeze all the roast garlic out into a small bowl and mash together with a fork. Spread the mashed garlic across the surface of the dough and top with one or two layers of grilled vegetables. Sprinkle with the Italian herbs, salt, and pepper.
- ▸ Roll up the bread (like rolling up a cinnamon roll) to form a long narrow loaf, pinching the seam and ends closed. Place on the prepared baking sheet. Brush the top of the loaf with a little water and sprinkle with poppy seeds.
- ▸ Bake 30 minutes, until the loaf is nicely browned. Allow to cool before slicing.

VARIATION: Feel free to substitute other grilled vegetables, such as bell peppers strips, onions, or thin slices of portobello mushroom, for the eggplant and zucchini. Just make sure that all vegetables are sliced thinly and grilled well. If your filling is too thick or too wet, you'll have a soggy Stromboli on your hands.

QUICK AND EASY VARIATION 1: Use prepackaged pizza or bread dough from the store.

QUICK AND EASY VARIATION 2: Substitute vegan turkey or ham deli slices and slices of vegan cheese for the grilled vegetables and roasted garlic.

Allergen Information * Soy-free, nut-free. Contains gluten and wheat.

MINI BURGER BUNS

This dough also makes great regular-size buns, dinner rolls, or veggie dog buns; simply change the shape and size and adjust the baking time accordingly.

Makes 12 to 13 buns

----
1 package (2¼ teaspoons) active dry yeast

2 tablespoons sugar

1 cup warm nondairy milk (110°F)

⅛ cup canola oil

½ teaspoon kosher salt

3–3½ cups all-purpose flour

▸ Warm ¼ cup water to 110°F (the water should be warm to the touch but not scalding—too hot and it will kill the yeast). Sprinkle the yeast and a pinch of the sugar into the warm water, stirring constantly. Let the mixture sit for 5 minutes to dissolve the yeast.

▸ Stir the warm nondairy milk, oil, the rest of the sugar, the salt, and the yeast mixture together in a mixing bowl. Add the flour cup by cup, stirring with a wooden spoon until the dough begins to form a ball.

▸ Turn the dough out onto a lightly floured surface and knead. As you knead, add enough extra flour to keep the dough from sticking. Knead for about 10 minutes, until the dough is smooth, elastic, and supple.

▸ Place the dough in a well-oiled mixing bowl, turning to cover the top of the dough with some of the oil. Cover with plastic wrap and a kitchen towel and place in a warm, draft-free place to rise until doubled in bulk, about 1 hour.

▸ Preheat oven to 375°F. Line a baking sheet with parchment paper, spray with nonstick spray, and set aside.

- Turn the dough out onto a lightly floured surface and press flat. Use a knife to cut the dough into 12 or 13 equal pieces. Roll each piece into a smooth ball and press each ball into a flat circle, about 2½ or 3 inches in diameter and ½ inch thick. Place the buns on the prepared baking sheet about 2 inches apart.
- Spray or brush the buns with oil and drape loosely with plastic wrap and let the buns rise for 30 minutes.
- Bake 12 minutes, or until golden. Set the buns on a wire rack to cool.

QUICK AND EASY VARIATION: If you don't have time to bake but still want miniature burger buns, use store-bought dinner rolls instead. Cut out part of the middle of the roll if necessary so they aren't too thick.

Allergen ✳ Information   Soy-free, nut-free. Contains gluten and wheat.

MINI PITA BREAD

(The Middle East)

Making your own pita bread is actually easier than you might think. The flatbreads bake quickly on a preheated baking (pizza) stone.

Makes 12 pitas

1½ cups warm water (110°F)

1 package (2¼ teaspoons) active dry yeast

1 teaspoon sugar

1 cup whole wheat flour

2 cups white bread flour, plus more for
   kneading and rolling

1½ teaspoons kosher salt

2 tablespoons olive oil

▸ Place the warm water in a mixing bowl and sprinkle with the yeast and sugar, stirring well. Let the mixture sit for 5 minutes to dissolve the yeast.

▸ In another bowl whisk together the whole wheat flour, 2 cups bread flour, and salt. Add the olive oil to the yeast mixture, and then stir the yeast mixture continually as you add in the flour cup by cup.

▸ When the flour mixture is incorporated and the dough begins to form a ball, turn the dough out onto a lightly floured surface and knead. As you knead, add enough extra flour to keep the dough from sticking. Knead for about 10 to 12 minutes, until the dough is smooth, elastic, and supple.

▸ Place the dough in a well-oiled mixing bowl, turning to cover the top of the dough with some of the oil. Cover with plastic wrap and a kitchen towel, and place in a warm, draft-free place to rise until doubled in bulk, about 1 hour.

- ▸ Place a baking (pizza) stone in the oven and preheat to 475°F.
- ▸ Turn the dough out onto a lightly floured surface and press flat. Use a knife to cut the dough into 12 equal pieces. Roll each piece into a smooth ball and place on a lightly floured surface. Cover the dough balls with plastic wrap and let the dough rest for 15 minutes.
- ▸ On a lightly floured surface use a rolling pin to roll each ball into a flat circle, about 4½ inches in diameter and ¼ inch thick.
- ▸ Bake the pitas directly on the heated baking stone for 3 minutes, or until puffed and golden brown. Set the pitas on a wire rack to cool.

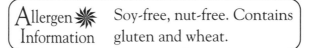

Allergen Information — Soy-free, nut-free. Contains gluten and wheat.

NAAN (INDIAN FLATBREAD)

(India)

These tender flatbreads are traditionally cooked on the sides of an extremely hot clay oven called a *tandoor*. I've found I get closest to replicating the taste and texture of restaurant naan when I cook my naan outside on a hot charcoal grill. For convenience, I've written this recipe with indoor baking instructions, but if you feel like firing up an outdoor grill you can brush both sides of the naan with oil and cook them directly on the hot grill.

Makes 8
small naan

1 cup warm nondairy milk (110°F)

1 teaspoon sugar

2¼ teaspoons (1 package) active dry yeast

2 tablespoons canola oil

2½ cups all-purpose flour, plus more as needed

1 teaspoon kosher salt

Nonhydrogenated margarine, melted (optional)

▶ Place the warm nondairy milk and sugar in a medium mixing bowl. Sprinkle with the yeast, stirring to dissolve. Let the mixture sit for 5 minutes to dissolve the yeast.

▶ Add the oil, 2 cups of the flour, and salt. Stir to combine, then add as much additional flour as needed to form a cohesive dough. Turn the dough out onto a lightly floured surface. Knead until smooth and elastic, about 10 minutes, adding flour as necessary to keep the dough from sticking. Place the dough in a well-oiled mixing bowl, turning to cover the top of the dough with some of the oil. Cover with plastic wrap and a kitchen towel and place in a warm, draft-free place to rise for about 1 hour.

- ▶ Toward the end of rising time, place a baking stone (pizza stone) in the oven and preheat to 500°F.
- ▶ Turn the dough out onto a lightly floured surface and divide into eight equal pieces. Use a rolling pin and/or your hands to flatten and pull each piece into a thin circle, about ⅛ inch thick.
- ▶ Bake the naan directly on the heated baking stone, flipping once halfway through, about 1½ minutes per side. (Press the naan down with a spatula if they start to inflate like pita bread.) Remove from the oven and brush with melted nonhydrogenated margarine if desired.

Allergen ✳ Information   Soy-free, nut-free. Contains gluten and wheat.

FRUIT SIDES

APPLE BUNNIES

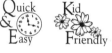

(Japan)

In Japanese these are called *usagi ringo* (*usagi* = rabbit, *ringo* = apple).
They are apple slices cut to resemble a rabbit with long ears.

1 apple makes 8 rabbits	1 lemon
	1 large, thick-skinned apple (such as a Fuji)

▸ Squeeze the lemon juice into a small bowl and fill the bowl with cold water. Set aside.

▸ Cut the apple into eight slices. Cut out the center core of each slice with a sharp paring knife.

▸ Use the sharp knife to cut a V shape into one end of the apple slice with the point of the V in the middle of the apple, cutting just through the skin and not all the way through the flesh. Carefully pare away the apple skin inside the V, removing the peel and revealing the flesh underneath. The two points of peel that are left on either side are the bunny's ears.

▸ Slip your knife under the "ears" and separate them from the flesh so they point out. Immerse the finished bunny in the lemon water for a minute or two so it doesn't turn brown in the lunch box.

Allergen ✳ Information   Gluten-free, wheat-free, soy-free, nut-free.

APPLESAUCE

Nothing could be easier than making your own applesauce. The variations are almost endless: leave it chunky or whir it smooth, add cinnamon or leave it plain, add pears or puréed berries, and so on. Sweet apples make a sweet applesauce; apples like Granny Smiths will make it tarter. My favorite applesauce combo is five Golden Delicious apples and one Granny Smith.

Makes about
4 cups

6 medium apples, peeled, cored, and cut
    into chunks
¼ cup golden raisins
½ cup apple juice or water
1 teaspoon cinnamon (optional)
1 to 2 teaspoons freshly squeezed
    lemon juice (optional)

▸ Place the apples, golden raisins, and apple juice in a medium saucepan and bring to a boil. Lower the heat and simmer, covered, until the apples are very tender, about 20 minutes.

▸ Cool slightly, then mash with a potato masher for a chunky applesauce, or process in a food processor fitted with the S blade for a smooth applesauce.

▸ Stir in cinnamon if you like. If your apples are very sweet you may wish to add some lemon juice to bring the flavor up and add a touch of tartness.

VARIATIONS: Add some puréed, strained berries (raspberries, strawberries, blueberries, etc.) to change the color and flavor of your applesauce. Substitute a pear or two for some of the apples.

Allergen Information ✳ Gluten-free, wheat-free, soy-free, nut-free.

BALSAMIC STRAWBERRIES

You can make cheap, watery balsamic vinegar from the grocery store taste like expensive, well-aged *balsamico* by reducing it a bit on the stovetop. Add a touch of sugar and lemon and you have a wonderful topping for fruit.

Makes 4 servings

½ cup balsamic vinegar

3 tablespoons sugar

1½ teaspoons freshly squeezed lemon juice

2 pounds (about 4 cups) fresh strawberries, hulled and halved

▸ Combine the vinegar and sugar in a small saucepan (note: don't use an aluminum saucepan for this one or the taste will be off). Bring to a boil over high heat and simmer until syrupy and reduced by half, about 5 minutes.

▸ Pour the balsamic mixture into a small bowl and add the lemon juice. Allow to cool completely (the syrup can be made a day ahead and stored in the refrigerator).

▸ Drizzle cooled syrup over the strawberries.

Allergen ☀ Information   Gluten-free, wheat-free, soy-free, nut-free.

LIMEADE FRUIT SALAD

My aunt Teresa brought this pretty fruit salad to a family meal, and I was immediately smitten. Thawed frozen limeade makes the watermelon and honeydew come alive.

Makes 4 servings

½ cup agave nectar

½ cup thawed frozen limeade concentrate

1 tablespoon poppy seeds

3 cups watermelon balls

3 cups honeydew melon balls

2 cups green grapes

▸ Mix the agave, limeade concentrate, and poppy seeds in a large mixing bowl. Carefully toss the fruit with the agave mixture.

Allergen Information ✳ Gluten-free, wheat-free, soy-free, nut-free.

MEXICAN FRUIT SALAD

(Mexico)

This colorful fruit salad mixes jicama and cucumber together with tropical fruit. Ancho chile powder gives the dish a sweet warmth. If you can't find it, substitute paprika and a pinch of cayenne.

Makes 6 servings

---
2 ripe mangoes (about 2 cups), peeled
    and diced
2 cups watermelon, cut into bite-size pieces
2 cups fresh pineapple, diced
1 cup jicama, peeled and cut into
    bite-size pieces
1 cup cucumber, peeled, quartered, and cut
    into bite-size pieces
Juice of 1 orange (about ½ cup)
Juice of 2 limes (about ¼ cup)
2 tablespoons sugar
Pinch of salt
1 teaspoon dried ancho chile powder
    (or ¾ teaspoon paprika mixed with
    ¼ teaspoon cayenne)

▸ Place the mango, watermelon, pineapple, jicama, and cucumber in a large mixing bowl.

▸ Mix the orange juice, lime juice, sugar, and salt together in a small bowl. Stir well, then pour over the fruit and toss gently. Sprinkle with the ancho chile powder.

Allergen ✳ Information Gluten-free, wheat-free, soy-free, nut-free.

ORANGES WITH RASPBERRY SAUCE AND PICKLED GINGER

This is a nice way to add excitement to oranges in the middle of winter, when most other fruits are out of season. Pickled ginger adds just the right touch of zing.

Makes 4 servings

6 large oranges

One 10-ounce package frozen raspberries, thawed

Sugar, to taste (optional)

¼ cup finely sliced pickled ginger

▶ Peel and segment the oranges and remove all the membrane (I cheat on this and cut my oranges in half, then score and scoop them out just like a grapefruit). Do this over a medium bowl to collect all the extra juice. Place the orange segments into another large bowl.

▶ Put all the extra juice into a blender along with the thawed frozen raspberries. Blend until smooth. Taste and add a little sugar if desired.

▶ Divide the orange segments into four bowls and top with a generous amount of pickled ginger. Serve with raspberry sauce.

Allergen ✳ Information — Gluten-free, wheat-free, soy-free, nut-free.

PEACHES PRALINE

Kid Friendly

This praline topping is perfect on freshly sliced peaches or baked apples.

> Makes about
> 2 cups

2 tablespoons cornstarch

¾ cup soy creamer

½ cup nonhydrogenated margarine

2 cups brown sugar

1 teaspoon vanilla

½ cup chopped pecans

Fresh peaches

▸ Dissolve the cornstarch in a bit of the soy creamer and stir until smooth. Set aside.

▸ Melt the margarine in a medium saucepan over medium-high heat. Add the brown sugar, soy creamer, and cornstarch mixture. Bring the mixture to a boil, stirring frequently. Boil for two minutes, stirring or whisking constantly.

▸ Remove from the heat and stir in the vanilla and pecans. Refrigerate the sauce until completely cool (the sauce will thicken as it cools).

▸ To serve, peel and slice peaches and top each serving with praline sauce. Store any unused sauce in the refrigerator.

Allergen Information ✳ Gluten-free, wheat-free. Contains soy, nuts, and corn.

STEWED APRICOTS

I love to snack on these tender, sweet apricots right out of the refrigerator. They also make a wonderful topping for hot cooked cereal in the morning.

Makes 1 cup

1 cup dried apricots

½ cup orange juice

▸ Place the apricots and orange juice in a small saucepan and bring to a boil over high heat. Turn off the heat, cover the pan, and let the apricots stew until tender and plump but not mushy, about 5 to 10 minutes. Note that you may have to increase the soaking time or even simmer the apricots for 1 to 2 minutes before turning off the heat if you are using very dry unsulphured apricots.
▸ Transfer the apricots and juice to a covered container and store in the refrigerator.

Allergen Information — Gluten-free, wheat-free, soy-free, nut-free.

STUFFED DATES

Quick & Easy

What a simple, natural dessert these are! They look lovely arranged along the edges of a fruit platter at a party. Use large, soft, pitted dates like Medjools or Deglet Noors.

Makes 12 dates

12 whole pitted dates

6 teaspoons almond butter

12 whole almonds, toasted or raw

▶ Use a small sharp knife to cut open each date along one side. Press the dates gently open and stuff each with ½ teaspoon almond butter. Press a whole almond into the top of each date.

VARIATIONS: Replace the whole almonds with pecan or walnut halves.

Allergen ❋ Information Gluten-free, wheat-free, soy-free. Contains nuts.

TROPICAL FRUIT SALAD

When I make fresh fruit salads for the lunch box, I usually slice the fruit into large chunks and leave grapes and berries whole, so my son can eat the salad one fruit at a time if he prefers. Sadly, this also means he can pick up the fruit chunks and eat them with his fingers (it's shocking what some kids will do to get lunch over with fast and go to recess).

This salad is a bit different: each fruit is diced into tiny pieces, so that the flavor of every fruit is present in each bite. This is one fruit salad that even my son has to eat with a spoon.

Makes 4 servings

1 cup fresh pineapple spears

½ medium fresh papaya, peeled and seeded

1 medium fresh mango, peeled and cut away from the pit

1 cup green grapes

4 tablespoons full-fat coconut milk or coconut cream

▸ Dice each of the fruits into small pieces, about ⅛ inch. Mix the fruits together in a large mixing bowl.

▸ To serve, divide the fruit salad into four bowls and top each serving with a spoonful of coconut milk.

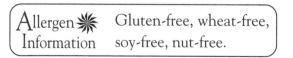

Allergen Information — Gluten-free, wheat-free, soy-free, nut-free.

DESSERTS

BROWN SUGAR SHORTBREAD

Shortbread cookies are a traditional cookie from Scotland. This version is made with brown sugar rather than white, changing them to a pretty brown color and adding flavor. Shortbread flavor is all about butter, so use the best-tasting nondairy margarine you can find (I like Earth Balance). These cookies keep well and taste even better when they are cool, making them excellent gifts.

Makes about 20
2-inch cookies

½ cup nonhydrogenated margarine, at
    room temperature
¼ cup plus 2 tablespoons packed
    brown sugar
1 cup all-purpose flour plus more for rolling
    out the dough

▸ Cream the margarine and brown sugar together with a hand-held mixer or a stand mixer fitted with the paddle attachment until light and creamy. Add the flour and mix together by hand until a dough forms. Form the dough into a 1-inch thick disk, wrap in plastic wrap, and refrigerate for one hour.

▸ Dust your working surface with flour and roll the dough out ¼ inch thick. Cut cookies out with a knife or cookie cutters. Place the cookies 1 inch apart on an ungreased cookie sheet and freeze for one hour.

▸ Preheat oven to 300°F. Bake until cookies are set but not hard or browned, about 20 minutes. Cool on a wire rack. (Shortbread cookies taste better a day or two after they are made.)

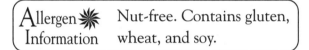

Allergen Information — Nut-free. Contains gluten, wheat, and soy.

CHOCOLATE BABKA MUFFINS

Babka is made from bread dough twisted around a filling of chocolate and cinnamon and topped with streusel. Normally it's baked in a loaf, but after I read that Barney Greengrass on Manhattan's Upper West Side makes individual babkas baked in muffin tins, I had to give it a try for my New York lunch box.

Makes 12 muffins

----

1 recipe Mini Burger Bun dough (page 196)

For the filling:
1 cup vegan chocolate chips, ground in
    a food processor until finely chopped
½ teaspoon cinnamon
2½ tablespoons sugar
2 tablespoons nonhydrogenated margarine,
    at room temperature

For the streusel topping:
1½ tablespoons all-purpose flour
1½ tablespoons sugar
¼ teaspoon cinnamon
1 tablespoon nonhydrogenated margarine

▸ Follow the instructions for preparing, kneading, and rising the bread dough.

▸ While the dough is on its first rise, line 12 muffin cups with paper liners and spray the muffin papers with nonstick spray (otherwise the muffins will stick). Set aside.

▸ Make the chocolate filling by combining the ground chocolate chips, cinnamon, sugar, and margarine in a mixing bowl. Knead the mixture together with a spoon or your hands until the margarine is completely incorporated.

- In a separate mixing bowl, make the streusel topping by combining the flour, sugar, cinnamon, and margarine, working the margarine in until well combined and crumbly. Turn the dough out onto a lightly floured surface. Press the air bubbles out and use a lightly floured rolling pin to roll the dough out into a 12 x 14-inch rectangle. Spread the dough evenly with the chocolate filling, leaving a small strip of dough uncovered at one end.
- Roll the dough up like a cinnamon roll, rolling toward the uncovered edge. Pinch the ends closed, using a bit of water brushed along the uncovered surface to help it seal. Cut the roll into twelve equal pieces and place each piece in a prepared muffin cup.
- Crumble the streusel evenly on top of the muffins. Let the muffins rest for about 10 minutes while you preheat the oven to 350°F. Bake muffins for 20 to 25 minutes, until golden brown. Let cool for several minutes before removing from the pan. Cool on a wire rack.

Allergen ✳ Information — Nut-free. Contains gluten, wheat, and soy.

COCONUT CREAM PIELETTES

These little coconut pies are sturdy enough to travel well in a lunch box or picnic basket.

Look in the baking section at your grocery store for vegan-friendly ready-made graham cracker piecrusts. Keebler makes mini graham cracker piecrusts in packages of six. If your store doesn't carry the small ones, this recipe makes enough to fill one regular size graham cracker piecrust instead.

Makes 6
small pies

⅓ cup sweet flake coconut, toasted
   (see below)
6 ounces soft silken tofu
⅓ cup sugar
5 tablespoons cornstarch
1 (14-ounce) can light coconut milk
1 teaspoon vanilla
⅛ teaspoon coconut extract
6 mini graham cracker piecrusts

▶ To toast coconut, preheat the oven to 350°F, spread the coconut out in a thin layer on a baking sheet, and toast, stirring or shaking the pan occasionally, until the coconut is golden, about 5 minutes.

▶ In a blender, blend the silken tofu until smooth and set aside. In a medium saucepan whisk together the sugar and cornstarch. Add the coconut milk and cook over medium-high heat, stirring or whisking constantly, until thick, about 7 to 8 minutes. Remove from heat, then fold in the tofu, vanilla, coconut extract, and shredded coconut. Divide evenly into the mini graham piecrusts and chill.

Allergen ✳ Information   Nut-free. Contains gluten, wheat, and soy.

EASY VEGAN SPONGE CAKE

If you're making this for Lamingtons (page 224), bake it a day ahead of time and refrigerate. This is also a good cake to serve plain or topped with jam or fresh strawberries.

Makes 12 squares

2 cups all-purpose flour

4 teaspoons baking powder

½ teaspoon baking soda

¼ teaspoon salt

1 teaspoon apple cider vinegar

6 tablespoons nonhydrogenated margarine,
    at room temperature

¾ cup sugar

1 teaspoon vanilla extract

▸ Preheat the oven to 350°F. Spray a 9 x 9-inch pan with nonstick spray and line with parchment paper. Spray the parchment paper with nonstick spray. Set aside.

▸ In a medium mixing bowl, whisk together the flour, baking powder, baking soda, and salt. Combine 1 cup water with the vinegar in a liquid measuring cup. Set aside.

▸ Cream together the margarine, sugar, and vanilla in a mixing bowl with a handheld electric mixer or in a stand mixer using the paddle attachment.

▸ Alternately add the water mixture and the flour mixture to the mixing bowl, beginning and ending with water. Beat until smooth and well blended, stopping to scrape down the sides as needed.

▸ Pour the cake batter into the prepared pan. Bake for 25 minutes, until a cake tester or toothpick inserted into the center comes out clean.

▸ Cool in the pan for 15 to 20 minutes, then turn the cake out to cool completely on a wire rack, removing the parchment paper.

Allergen ✳ Information   Nut-free. Contains gluten, wheat, and soy.

GLORIFIED RICE

I grew up eating sweet, fluffy Glorified Rice at my Grandma's house each Thanksgiving and Christmas. Grandma and Betty Crocker taught me to mix rice with crushed pineapple, whipped cream, and maraschino cherries. But now that so many people in our family are vegan and more health-conscious, I wanted to come up with a nondairy version without the neon cherries. I did it! The flavor is so spot-on, even Grandma approves!

Makes 6 to 8 servings	1 cup dry short grain white rice 1 20-ounce can crushed pineapple, well drained ½ cup plus 4 tablespoons sugar 1 12.3-ounce package firm silken tofu 2 tablespoons fresh lemon juice 1 pint fresh strawberries, rinsed, topped, and sliced

▸ Cook the white rice according to package directions. While the rice is still hot, place the rice in a large mixing bowl and stir in the crushed pineapple and ½ cup sugar. Let the mixture rest at room temperature for one hour to cool. Cover and refrigerate until cold.

▸ Place the silken tofu, 4 tablespoons sugar, and lemon juice in a blender. Blend until completely smooth. Fold the blended tofu into the rice mixture, breaking apart any clumps of rice with a wooden spoon. Top with freshly sliced strawberries and serve.

Allergen ✳ Information — Gluten-free, wheat-free, nut-free. Contains soy.

JIGGLEGELS

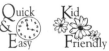

One of the biggest shocks I had when I first turned vegetarian was discovering where gelatin came from: the boiled bones, skins, and tendons of animals. Yuck!

But worry not! I hereby give you JiggleGels: all-natural, all-vegan, sugar-free gel snacks. The secret is agar agar, a gelling powder derived from seaweed. Look for agar agar powder at health food stores or online at sites like Amazon.com.

Makes 4 cups

4 cups 100% juice fruit punch

2 teaspoons agar agar powder

▶ If you wish to cut the JiggleGels into squares or shapes, have a 10 x 15-inch jellyroll pan with a raised edge standing by. If you wish to mold it or simply eat it with a spoon, have ready any gelatin molds (sprayed with nonstick spray), bowls, or lunch box containers you prefer.

▶ Bring the juice to a boil in a medium saucepan. Sprinkle the agar agar powder over the top, whisking constantly. The juice will foam up when the powder hits it, but will subside again in a minute or so. Boil for 3 minutes, whisking frequently.

▶ Pour the liquid into the pan or bowls (sometimes I end up with a couple bits of agar agar that did not dissolve; if this happens to you, pour the liquid through a fine sieve). Place carefully in the refrigerator and refrigerate until completely set, about one hour.

▶ Cut the gelled juice into squares or use cookie cutters to cut out fun shapes, removing them from the pan with a thin spatula.

VARIATIONS: Use any juice you like to make different flavors and colors of gel. You can also add sliced fresh or canned fruit to the gel before it is completely set.

┌───┐
│ Allergen ✳ Gluten-free, wheat-free,   │
│ Information   soy-free, nut-free.   │
└───┘

LAMINGTONS

(Australia)

Chocolate-dipped, coconut-covered Lamingtons were invented in Queensland, Australia, as a way to reinvent stale sponge cake. They were named after Lady Lamington, the wife of the Governor of Queensland in the late 1800s.

Use heated leftover chocolate icing to dip Brown Sugar Shortbread (page 215) or spread room temperature icing with a knife onto fresh fruit or vegan graham crackers.

Makes 12 Lamingtons

----
1 recipe Easy Vegan Sponge Cake
    (page 220), made at least one day
    ahead and refrigerated
2 cups finely shredded sweetened or
    desiccated coconut
4 cups powdered sugar
½ cup cocoa powder
½ cup nondairy milk
2 tablespoons nonhydrogenated margarine
1½ teaspoons vanilla

- Cut the sponge cake into twelve 2¼ x 3-inch squares.
- Place the coconut in a large shallow bowl. Set aside.
- To make the chocolate icing, sift the powdered sugar and cocoa powder together in a medium bowl; set aside. In a small saucepan, heat the nondairy milk and margarine to a boil over medium-high heat. Transfer to the top of a double boiler or a heat-proof bowl over a pan of simmering water. Add the powdered sugar/cocoa mixture and the vanilla. Whisk until completely smooth. Keep the icing over simmering water as you work to keep it soft.
- Dip each cake into the icing, using two forks to help turn and coat all sides. Hold the dripping cake aloft and let the excess icing drip off. Now use two more forks to roll the cake in coconut. Transfer to a wire rack and repeat with the remaining cakes.
- Let the icing set for about 15 minutes, then transfer to a covered container and keep refrigerated until ready to serve.

Allergen ❋ Information   Nut-free. Contains gluten, wheat, and soy.

MINI VEGAN CHEESECAKES

These muffin-size cheesecakes are baked in foil cupcake liners, making them easy to pop into a lunch box. Pack some fresh berries alongside to top the cheesecakes with at lunchtime.

Makes 12 mini cheesecakes

1 cup vegan graham cracker crumbs

4 tablespoons maple syrup or Frugal Momma's "Maple" Syrup (page 60)

16 ounces vegan cream cheese

¾ cup sugar

3 tablespoons lemon juice

1½ teaspoons vanilla

3 tablespoons all-purpose flour

Berries or other fruit for topping, if desired

▸ Preheat the oven to 350°F. Line 12 muffin cups with foil cupcake liners and set aside.

▸ To make the crust, mix together the graham cracker crumbs and maple syrup. Spoon a bit more than 1 tablespoon of crumbs into each cupcake liner. Use a tart tamper or the bottom of a glass to press the crumbs to the bottom firmly.

▸ Blend together the vegan cream cheese, sugar, lemon juice, and vanilla until creamy, using a handheld mixer or the bowl of a stand mixer fitted with the paddle attachment. Fold in the flour and mix to combine.

▸ Divide the mixture evenly into the prepared muffin cups (about ⅓ cup in each). Bake for 20 to 25 minutes or until puffed and dry on top. Cool on a wire rack (the cheesecakes will deflate a bit as they cool). Remove from the muffin pan and refrigerate several hours or overnight.

▸ Top with berries or other fruit, if desired.

> Allergen ✳ Information | Nut-free. Contains gluten, wheat, and soy.

OATMEAL COOKIES

A sweet, simple vegan cookie for the lunch box, made nut-, wheat-, and soy-free so even children with multiple allergies can enjoy them. Oatmeal cookies also make a nice after-school snack with a glass of nondairy milk.

Makes 3 dozen cookies

¾ cup canola oil

1 cup packed brown sugar

1 cup white sugar

½ cup plain nondairy milk

2 teaspoons vanilla

2½ cups barley flour

1 teaspoon baking powder

1 teaspoon baking soda

1 teaspoon kosher salt

2 cups quick rolled oats (or old-fashioned rolled oats pulsed in a food processor)

½ cup raisins

- Preheat oven to 350°F. Line a baking sheet with parchment paper and spray with nonstick spray. Set aside.
- Cream together the oil, brown sugar, and white sugar in a mixing bowl using a handheld mixer or in the bowl of a stand mixer fitted with the paddle attachment. Add the nondairy milk and vanilla and beat to combine.
- Meanwhile, sift together the flour, baking powder, baking soda, and salt. Add to the sugar mixture and beat to combine. At this point the cookie dough will be quite stiff, so use a wooden spoon or your hands to add the oats and raisins and mix well.
- Using a 1-ounce cookie scoop or a large spoon, place scoops of cookie dough on the baking sheet about 3 inches apart. Flatten and shape the cookies gently with your hands.
- Bake until golden brown around the edges, about 14 to 15 minutes. Transfer the cookies to a wire rack to cool.

VARIATIONS: Add ½ cup chopped nuts, if you like. Substitute ½ cup chopped dates for the raisins.

Allergen Information ✳ Wheat-free, soy-free, nut-free. Contains gluten.

PRICKLY PEAR PUDDING

(Southwestern United States)

Make this simple stove-top pudding the night before, pouring it directly into a small lunch box container and putting it in the refrigerator. In the morning your pudding will be ready to go.

Prickly pears are the bright red fruit of the nopale cactus. Prickly pear syrup turns this pudding a delicious shade of pink. Look for prickly pear syrup at specialty stores or online at www.desertusa.com.

Makes 4 servings

4 tablespoons cornstarch

2 cups nondairy milk

4 tablespoons sugar

2 tablespoons prickly pear syrup, plus more
   for serving, if desired

▶ Place the cornstarch in a small bowl and slowly pour in about ½ cup of the nondairy milk, whisking constantly with a fork or small whisk. Whisk until the cornstarch is completely dissolved, then set aside.

▶ Pour the remaining nondairy milk into a medium saucepan. Stir in the sugar and heat the mixture on medium, stirring frequently, until the mixture begins to steam and looks close to boiling.

▶ Add the cornstarch mixture and immediately begin stirring constantly. Stir with a wooden spoon or whisk until the mixture comes to a boil and thickens to a pudding consistency. This will take at least 1 to 2 minutes after boiling begins (cornstarch needs to boil for at least one minute in order to start thickening).

▶ Turn off the heat and add the prickly pear syrup, stirring until the pudding is a uniform pink. Pour the pudding into four dessert bowls or lunch box containers. Refrigerate for several hours or overnight.

▸ Serve with more prickly pear syrup on the side to pour over the top, if desired.

VARIATION: If you don't have any prickly pear syrup handy, substitute any fruit-flavored syrup you like—blackberry, strawberry, and so on.

Allergen ✳ Information   Gluten-free, wheat-free, soy-free, nut-free. Contains corn.

RUSSIAN TEA CAKES

(Russia)

These simple cookies look like little snowballs. Use your favorite kind of jam to make them. We like seedless raspberry.

Makes 24 tea cakes	½ cup nonhydrogenated margarine, at room temperature
	3 tablespoons jam
	1 tablespoon plus ⅓ cup powdered sugar
	1 cup plus 1 tablespoon all-purpose flour
	3 tablespoons finely chopped or ground walnuts (optional)

▸ Preheat oven to 325°F. Line a baking sheet with parchment paper, spray with nonstick spray, and set aside.

▸ Cream the margarine, jam, and 1 tablespoon powdered sugar together in a mixing bowl using a handheld mixer, or in the bowl of a stand mixer using the paddle attachment.

▸ Add the cup and tablespoon of flour and the walnuts, if using, and blend well. Use your hands to roll bits of dough into 24 1-inch balls. Place the cookies one inch apart on the prepared baking sheet (add a bit more flour if necessary to stiffen the dough so it can be shaped into balls).

▸ Bake 18 to 20 minutes, until firm to the touch and golden brown on the bottom. Cool completely on a wire rack.

▸ When the tea cakes are completely cool, place the remaining ⅓ cup powdered sugar in a small bowl and roll the cookies to completely cover them in sugar.

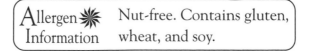

Allergen Information ✳ Nut-free. Contains gluten, wheat, and soy.

SPITZBUBEN (LITTLE RASCALS)

Kid Friendly

(Germany)

These pretty sandwich cookies filled with jam are sure to keep your little rascals happy! Spitzbuben are best baked and filled a day ahead of time.

Makes 24 cookies

1 cup sugar

¾ cup nonhydrogenated margarine

1 teaspoon almond extract

2 cups all-purpose flour

½ cup almond meal or ground almonds
(process blanched almonds or almond
slivers in a food processor)

¼ cup of your favorite jam or jelly

▸ Cream together the sugar, margarine, and almond extract with a handheld mixer or stand mixer fitted with the paddle attachment. Add the flour and almonds and mix well. Add 1 to 2 tablespoons water as needed to form a dough that holds together.

▸ Press the dough into a 1-inch thick disk. Wrap and chill the dough for one hour.

▸ Preheat the oven to 350°F. Line two baking sheets with parchment paper, spray with nonstick spray, and set aside.

▸ Roll the dough out on a lightly floured surface to ⅛ inch thick. Cut out 48 2-inch circles with a cookie cutter. Take half the cookies and cut a small circle or other shape out of the center with a small cookie cutter (these will be the tops of the sandwich cookies).

- ▸ Place the cookies 1 inch apart on the prepared baking sheets and bake until lightly brown, about 12 minutes. Cool on a wire rack.
- ▸ When the cookies are completely cool, place ½ teaspoon of jam or jelly in the center of the first cookies, then top with the cookies with cut-out centers, so that the jam shows through. (These cookies taste better a day after they are made.)

Allergen ✳ Information Contains gluten, flour, soy, and nuts.

BEVERAGES

GRAPE SPORTS DRINK

Quick
&
Easy

When it comes to exercise, it's really not necessary to down a store-bought sports drink after every single soccer game or dance practice. Unless you or your child are serious athletes exercising under extreme conditions (i.e., heat, long hours, dehydrating illness), water and a snack will usually suffice. But if your budding sports legend still longs for a special beverage, try this.

Makes 2 servings	2 cups filtered water
	¾ cup grape juice
	½ tablespoon fresh lemon juice
	1 tablespoon light agave nectar
	Pinch of sea salt

▸ Combine all ingredients and refrigerate until needed. Shake before drinking.

VARIATION: Substitute any unsweetened fruit juice you like.

Allergen ✳ Information — Gluten-free, wheat-free, soy-free, nut-free.

For more information about vegan athletes and nutrition, check out *Thrive: The Vegan Nutrition Guide to Optimal Performance in Sports and Life* by professional Ironman triathlete and vegan, Brendan Brazier. His book offers up sound advice for athletes along with all-natural recipes for gels, sports drinks, smoothies, and bars.

ICED LEMONGRASS TISANE

A tisane is an herbal infusion. This crystal-clear lemongrass tisane tastes bright and refreshing.

Makes 2 servings

1 cup lemongrass leaves and stems,
   cut into 1½-inch segments

1–2 teaspoons agave nectar (optional)

▸ Bring 2 cups water to almost boiling. Pour the water over the lemongrass and steep for 7 minutes. Strain into a pitcher, add the agave, if desired, and stir to dissolve. Chill until completely cold and serve over ice.

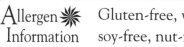

Allergen Information — Gluten-free, wheat-free, soy-free, nut-free.

LEMON-LIME SPARKLE

On average, a can of regular sweetened soda pop contains 10 teaspoons of sugar and 150 calories. Substitute some homemade sparkling water with just a splash of sweetness, and save those calories for some real food.

Makes 2 servings

1 tablespoon freshly squeezed lemon juice

1 tablespoon freshly squeezed lime juice

2–4 teaspoons agave nectar (more or less, to taste)

2 cups sparkling water (or regular water)

▸ Combine the lemon juice, lime juice, and agave and stir until the agave has blended in. Add the water, stir briefly, and chill. Serve with ice.

VARIATIONS: Substitute other unsweetened juices for the lemon and lime. Good combinations include pomegranate and lime; cranberry and pineapple; and blueberry and orange.

Allergen 🌟 Information   Gluten-free, wheat-free, soy-free, nut-free.

Carbonated soda is my *bête noire*. I will openly admit that I screwed up big time in introducing my toddler first to large servings of juice and then to soda pop. I didn't know then just how many empty, nutrition-free calories each soda and sweetened drink contained, or that the carbonation in soda actually causes our bodies to lose calcium.

Combine his early exposure with the power of advertising and his peers, and it's now become impossible to keep my son away from the stuff. He's always looking to nab a soda when he's out of the house. In addition, his growing involvement in team sports has convinced him that sweetened, colored "sports drinks" are the only way to rehydrate after an hour on the field.

If I had to do it over again, only water and calcium-fortified nondairy milks would be offered as regular daily beverages, with juices limited to use in whole fruit smoothies. Now all I can do is keep soda out of our house and offer these enjoyable, refreshing beverage options instead. I'm happy to say I've been making some headway! James especially loves my new Grape Sports Drink on page 235.

MEXICAN HOT CHOCOLATE

(Mexico)

Look for bars of cinnamon-flavored Mexican chocolate in the Mexican grocery section of the grocery stores. I use Ibarra brand.

Makes 3 to 4 servings

1 3-ounce disk of Mexican chocolate

2½ cups nondairy milk

▶ Chop the disk of Mexican chocolate and place it in a blender.

▶ Heat the nondairy milk in a medium saucepan over medium-high heat, stirring very frequently, until it comes to a boil.

▶ Immediately pour the hot milk into the blender and blend until the chocolate has melted into the milk and the mixture is frothy.

▶ Drink right away or pack this for a lunch by pouring the beverage into a preheated insulated food jar.

Allergen ✳ Information

Gluten-free, wheat-free, nut-free. Contains soy (soy lecithin in the Mexican chocolate).

PEACH SMOOTHIE

This was inspired by the incredible peach juice served at Nicholas Restaurant in Portland, Oregon. Their menu says it is "a popular juice enjoyed on almost every front porch in Lebanon." After tasting it, you'll understand why!

Makes 2 servings

½ cup peach juice, white grape peach juice, or other peach juice blend

½ cup soy creamer

1 cup frozen peaches

1 tablespoon freshly squeezed lemon juice

2 tablespoons almond-flavored syrup (the kind used for flavoring coffee drinks)

¼ teaspoon rose water (optional)

▸ Blend all ingredients until smooth.

Allergen ✳ Information   Gluten-free, wheat-free. Contains soy and nuts.

THAI ICED TEA

Thai Iced Tea is a beautiful drink to look at—creamy white at the top with swirls of cream dropping down into the brilliant orange tea below. I've replaced the traditional dairy cream in this recipe with rich coconut milk.

Thai tea is a special blend of tea leaves, anise, cinnamon, and vanilla. Look for it in Asian markets or online.

Makes 4 servings

2 tablespoons Thai tea

¼ cup sugar

8 tablespoons coconut milk or soy creamer

▸ Bring 4 cups of water to boil in a kettle or saucepan. (The flavor is best if you can catch the water before it comes to a large, rolling boil. The water should be "dancing.")

▸ Place the tea leaves in a bowl or large teapot (I use a large coffee press, so it's easy to strain the tea leaves out). Pour the water over the tea leaves and allow the tea to steep for 3 to 5 minutes (longer if you like strong tea).

▸ Strain the tea into a pitcher and add the sugar. Stir with a wooden spoon until the sugar is dissolved. Refrigerate until cold.

▸ To serve immediately, fill four ice tea glasses with ice cubes and pour in the tea, leaving an inch or so at the top of each glass. Add 2 tablespoons of coconut milk or soy creamer to each glass without stirring. Serve with straws and ice tea spoons, allowing each drinker to stir in the milk as they wish.

▸ To pack this tea in a lunch box, freeze some of the tea in an ice cube tray and use the frozen tea cubes in place of regular ice cubes. Your tea will stay cold without becoming watery in the lunch box. I like to pack the coconut cream separately and pour it in just before I drink it.

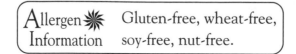

Allergen Information — Gluten-free, wheat-free, soy-free, nut-free.

VEGAN MARY

This is one of my favorite summertime beverages, served with one or two celery stalks for dipping and munching as I drink. Vegetarian Worcestershire sauce is available at health food stores and online (see the Recommended Resources section). Look for low-sodium tomato-vegetable juice blends at the grocery store; I recommend Knudsen's Very Veggie.

Makes 1 serving

----

4 ounces low-sodium tomato-vegetable juice
    or tomato juice

½ ounce freshly squeezed lemon juice

½ teaspoon vegetarian Worcestershire sauce

Dash of Tabasco sauce

Pinch of celery salt

Salt and freshly ground black pepper, to taste

Celery stalks and a lemon or lime wedge
    for garnish

▸ Shake all the ingredients except the garnishes together in a cocktail shaker filled with ice. Strain into a glass filled with ice (or pack without ice and add ice just before drinking). Garnish with celery stalks and a lemon or lime wedge.

Allergen ✳ Information   Gluten-free, wheat-free, soy-free, nut-free.

Recommended Resources

Books

Baer, Edith. *This Is the Way We Eat Our Lunch: A Book About Children Around the World*. New York: Scholastic, 1990.

A fun rhyming book to read to the younger set.

Grogan, Bryanna Clark. *Authentic Chinese Cuisine*. Summertown, TN: Book Publishing Company, 2000.

Vegan Chinese cooking by great chef and cookbook author Bryanna Clark Grogan. All of Bryanna's books are wonderful!

Jaffrey, Madhur. *Madhur Jaffrey's World Vegetarian: More Than 650 Meatless Recipes from Around the World*. New York: Clarkson Potter, 2002.

The book that opened my eyes to the amazing flavors of world vegetarian cuisine.

Manga University Culinary Institute. *The Manga Cookbook*. Japan: Japanime, 2007.

A cute introduction to Japanese cooking and bento packing, told by manga (Japanese comic book) characters.

McCann, Jennifer. *Vegan Lunch Box: 130 Amazing, Animal-Free Lunches Kids and Grown-Ups Will Love*. Cambridge, MA: Da Capo Press, 2008.

My first book! You'll find many more kid-friendly recipes here, all tested by my then seven-year-old son, along with well-balanced lunch menus, stories, pictures, and themed meals designed for seasonal holidays and special occasions. The book even includes more international cuisine, including lunch menus inspired by Mexico, Greece, Japan, England, India, Thailand, and France.

Pottle, Renee. *Homestyle Favorites Made Meatless: Cooking with Meat Substitutes*. Kennewick, WA: Hestia's Hearth, 2009.

Renee also makes and sells a great selection of vegan gourmet soup mixes; visit www.winebarrelgourmet.com.

Yuen, Susan. *Hawaii's Bento Box Cookbook: Fun Lunches for Kids*. Honolulu: Mutual Publishing, 2008.

Another inspirational book filled with Japanese bento. If you love to coo over lunches that look like teddy bears, princesses, and mermaids, this is the book for you. The recipes are not vegan; try substituting vegan deli slices and cheese and white veggies like jicama or daikon for the bologna, cheese, and fishcake in the designs.

Online Shopping

The Celtic Croft:www.kilts-n-stuff.com/Food_Products/haggis.htm

Vegetarian haggis and other Scottish accoutrement.

Copper Gifts: www.coppergifts.com

Copper cookie cutters in all sorts of shapes and sizes, including tiny fish-shaped cookie cutters for vegan fish crackers.

Eden Foods: www.edenfoods.com

A good source for all-natural Japanese foods, such as soba noodles, reduced sodium soy sauce, sea vegetables, and more.

Nature's Flavors: www.naturesflavors.com

All-natural vegan food colorings and flavors.

Pangea Vegan Store: www.veganstore.com

Look here for items like vegan Worcestershire sauce and vegan chicken- and beef-bouillon cubes.

Vegan Essentials: www.veganessentials.com

A fabulous source for all things vegan, including nondairy cheese crackers.

Lunch Boxes and Accessories

Bento TV: www.bentotv.com

Highly adorable short instructional videos on bento packing, free on-line, along with bento boxes and supplies.

I Love Obento!: www.iloveobento.com

Great selection of Japanese bento boxes and lunch box accessories. See insert page 4 (top), 8.

Laptop Lunches: www.laptoplunches.com

Home of the lunch box that started it all, the Laptop Lunch System, a wildly popular plastic American-style bento box. See insert page 3 (bottom), 8.

Lunchsense: www.lunchsense.com

An exciting new design out of Eugene, Oregon, featuring colorful carrying cases, multiple sizes to choose from, and tight snap-and-seal lids. See insert page 4 (bottom).

Pearl River: www.pearlriver.com

Colorful stacking melamine tiffins, stainless steel lunch boxes, and more. See insert page 1 (top), 7 (bottom), 8.

3GreenMoms: www.3greenmoms.com

If you use a lot of plastic sandwich bags in your lunches, try 3Green Mom's "Lunch Skins" instead—colorful cloth pouches that replace disposables.

Thermos: www.thermos.com

Insulated food jars and beverage bottles. See insert page 1 (bottom), 2, 7 (top).

To-Go Ware: www.to-goware.com

Stainless-steel tiffin-style lunch boxes. See insert page 5, 6 (bottom).

Index

mung bean sprouts
   Bean Sprout Salad, 75
   Vegetarian Pho, 103
   Zaru Soba, 136–137
Mung Dahl, 144–145
mushrooms
   Asian Portobellos, 161
   English Kidney (Bean) Pie,
      114–115
   Grilled Vegetable Stromboli
      (variation), 195
   Heavenly Mushrooms, 168
   New England Chowder, 99–100
   Roasted Veggie Kabobs, 178
   Vietnamese Salad Rolls, 91–92
   Zaru Soba, 136–137
My Favorite Tofurky Sandwich, 88

Naan (Indian Flatbread), 200–201
Nacho Cheese Dip, 63
navy beans, in Barbecue Baked Beans,
   142–143
Nebraskan menu, 5
New England Chowder, 99–100
New England menu, 6
New Orleans menu, 6–7
New York menu, 7
noodles
   Hot Noodle Soup, 93–94
   Mango Noodles, 124–125
   Noodles with Poppy Seeds, 147–148
   Vegetarian Pho, 103
   Vietnamese Salad Rolls, 91–92
   Zaru Soba, 136–137
Nopales, Fried, 167
nori
   California Roll, 110–111
   Zaru Soba, 136–137
nut butters
   African Greens, 157–158
   Jennifer's Omega-3 Protein Bars,
      55–56
   Stuffed Dates, 212

nutritional yeast flakes
   Chik'n Pot Pie, 113–114
   Mini Veggie Burgers, 126–127
   Nacho Cheese Dip, 63
nuts. *See specific types*

oat bran, in Cabbage Rolls,
   108–109
Oatmeal Cookies, 227–228
oats, in Mini Veggie Burgers,
   126–127
Octo-Celery, 71
okra, in Martie's Gumbo, 95–96
Okra, Oven-Roasted, 170
olives, in Banderillas, 68
Omega-3 Protein Bars, Jennifer's,
   55–56
Onigiri, 148–149
Onigiri Bento menu, 45
onions
   Banderillas, 68
   Kasha Kupecheskaya, 122–123
   Maui Onion Dip, 62
   Mujaddara, 128–129
   Thai Cucumber Salad, 84
orange juice and zest
   Mexican Fruit Salad, 208
   Orange Couscous, 150–151
   Sour Cream Scones, 192
   Stewed Apricots, 211
   Tzimmes, 186
Oranges with Raspberry Sauce and
   Pickled Ginger, 209
Oven-Roasted Okra, 170

Pad Thai, packaged mixes for, 38
Palak Paneer, 171–172
papaya, in Tropical Fruit Salad, 213
Paprikás, Chik'n, 112
Papusas, 129–130
parsley
   Cucumber Tomato Salad, 80
   Martie's Gumbo, 95–96